UNSAFE MOTHERHOOD

Fertility, Reproduction and Sexuality

For full volume listing, please see pages 252 and 253.

UNSAFE MOTHERHOOD
MAYAN MATERNAL MORTALITY AND
SUBJECTIVITY IN POST-WAR GUATEMALA

Nicole S. Berry

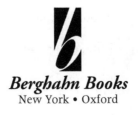

Berghahn Books
New York • Oxford

First published in 2010 by
Berghahn Books
www.BerghahnBooks.com

© 2010, 2013 Nicole S. Berry
First paperback edition published in 2013

Library of Congress Cataloging-in-Publication Data

Berry, Nicole S., 1970-
    Unsafe motherhood : Mayan maternal mortality and subjectivity in
post-war Guatemala / Nicole S. Berry.
        p. ; cm. — (Fertility, reproduction and sexuality, v. 21)
    Includes bibliographical references.
    ISBN 978-1-84545-752-5 (hbk.)--ISBN 978-0-85745-791-2 (pbk.)
    1. Mothers—Guatemala—Santa Cruz La Laguna—Mortality.
2. Pregnancy—Complications—Guatemala—Santa Cruz La Laguna.
3. Maternal health services—Guatemala—Santa Cruz La Laguna.
4. Childbirth at home—Guatemala—Santa Cruz La Laguna. I. Title.
II. Series: Fertility, reproduction, and sexuality, v. 21.
    [DNLM: 1. Maternal Welfare—ethnology—Guatemala.
2. Maternal Mortality—ethnology—Guatemala. 3. Prenatal Care—
Guatemala. WA 310 DG5 B534u 2010]
    RG530.3.G9B57 2010
    362.198'20097281—dc22
                                                        2010023812

British Library Cataloguing in Publication Data

A catalogue record for this book is available from the British Library.

Printed in the United States on acid-free paper

ISBN: 978-0-85745-791-2 (paperback)
eISBN: 978-0-85745-824-7 (retail ebook)

CONTENTS

List of Figures   vi

Acknowledgments   vii

Prologue. The Story of Rosario   xi

Introduction. The Specter of Death   1

Chapter 1. Life, Birth, and Death in the Village   23

Chapter 2. Coming to the ER: Analysis of an Interaction   60

Chapter 3. Global Safe Motherhood and Making Local
Pregnancy Safer: The Spin and What It Covers Up   85

Chapter 4. The Indio Bruto and Modern Guatemalan
Healthcare   108

Chapter 5. Everyday Violence: From a Kaqchikel Village to
the Nation and Back   130

Chapter 6. Praying for a Good Outcome: Staying at Home
during Obstetric Problems   160

Conclusion. Putting the "Maternal" Back in Maternal Mortality   190

Notes   196

Bibliography   219

Subject Index   236

Index to Ethnographic Vignettes   251

FIGURES

Illustrations

Illustration 1. Hospital birth in New Jersey, USA   9

Illustration 2. Homebirth in Atitlan, Guatemala   10

Illustration 3. The village of Santa Cruz   16

Illustration 4. Husband and wife collecting their catch in
Santa Cruz   27

Illustration 5. Weaver in Santa Cruz   28

Illustration 6. Woman hand stitching a huiple   29

Map

Map 1. Fieldsites in Sololá, Guatemala   17

Table

Table 1. History of previous birthing problems as a predictor
of actual difficulties   88

ACKNOWLEDGMENTS

My relationship with Guatemala and the choice of my field site have been personal as well as professional. I first traveled to Sololá with my father in the 1980s as a high school graduation present. The eeriness of a country in the midst of a civil war penetrated my teenage world and the things I remembered most about the country were the beauty, the violence, and the poverty. I returned to Guatemala in the summer of 1999 as a research assistant working in the Petén near the ruins of Tikal. Before I left the US a family friend gave me a key to her *casita* in Santa Cruz La Laguna, a hand-sketched map of the paths leading to her house, and urged me to take a vacation there since I was going to be so close. After the project in the Petén ended I traveled south to meet my boyfriend, who, as fate would have it, had been in Guatemala all summer doing a pilot study and looking for a field site. At the end of August we went to Santa Cruz and began to talk in earnest about how to continue our degrees and stay together. We stripped both of our projects down to their bare necessitates: I needed some sort of setting where clients interacted with a state agency, and he needed to work in an indigenous village of no less than 1,000 people. Though I wanted to work in Chile, it did not have a very extensive indigenous population. He wanted to work in a resettled Queqchi' village in the Petén, but I had spent my early twenties in the Peace Corps, living in an isolated village of 250 people without a telephone or any way to contact my friends or family, and repeating this experience in my 30s was not an idea that I savored. As a compromise we decided to investigate where we were. The next day we went to the Ministry of Health headquarters for Sololá to talk to the director about potential field sites in Sololá. No sooner had we introduced ourselves than he was telling us how much they needed a cultural anthropologist to do a study in the village of Santa Cruz, which had the highest levels of maternal mortality in the nation that year. The project fit my interests but, personally, I was more than happy to stay in Santa Cruz. The family friend who had given me the key, and who I had known since I was small child, now lived six months out of the year there. It was close to Panajachel, which had internet and telephone. And physically it was beautiful. Since choosing Santa Cruz as my field site my entire family has become more intertwined with the location. My father and stepmother built a house and now live there for five months of every year. My father's best friend, who lived with us throughout my childhood, and his partner followed. My husband and I also held our wedding ceremony there.

In a setting where family is a major social force, having these personal connections made my fieldwork easier for me. I felt like a legitimate social person because I, too, came as part of a group. Everyone knew me, they knew my husband, they knew my parents and my "aunts" and "uncle." My social responsibilities were parts of my life that easily translated. Without the presence of my family I would have been a disconnected, older, childless female who interviews people—a completely incomprehensible person. In addition, I'm not quite sure that I could have studied such an overwhelmingly depressing topic without the help of friends and family. Coming from the US, which is such an itinerant and age-segregated society, I do not know many of my friends' parents, my parents' friends' parents, or any of their grandparents. In other words, I have known very few people who have died. Dealing with death in Santa Cruz has been difficult for me as grieving in the village was an open process marked by much public crying and wailing. Public crying and wailing, however, do not comfort me. That my family has had some window into my research experience and thus some understanding of this part of my life has been invaluable to me.

This project has only been possible because I have benefited from the support and advice of many generous people and institutions. Several of them have been anonymous (reviewers) and I deeply appreciate the time and thought that they have put into providing me with feedback. Others I will list below, but there are still more who helped and will not be named because of confidentiality or space restrictions. I nevertheless remain in their debt.

The book began at the University of Michigan and could never have been possible without the help of various faculty members who taught me, questioned me, and engaged with what I had to say. I am particularly indebted to Bruce Mannheim, Larry Hirschfeld, and Fernando Coronil. I also thank Alaina Lemon, who agreed to step up to the plate at the last minute.

The Department of Anthropology, the Institute for Research on Women and Gender, and the Latin American Studies Program, all at the University of Michigan, Wenneren-Gren, and USED Fulbright-Hays provided the funding necessary to carry out my fieldwork, and I thank them for their support. I still would not have been able to complete this research without the generous help of many individuals and agencies in Guatemala. First, I would like to thank the Ministerio de Salud Pública y Asistencia Social, especially Dr. Nestor Carrillo-Poton and Dr. Mayron Martinez for their continual support and attention. Also, I would like to express my gratitude to Dr. Constantino Sánchez and Dr. Jorge Mendez for their invaluable assistance in providing me with access and cooperation in the hospital. Finally, Dr. Yadira Villaseñor de Cross of JHPIEGO oriented me in the campaign for Safe Motherhood in Sololá. Her constructive attitude and hard work on a difficult and sometimes depressing subject were inspiring. While I have perhaps too thoroughly embraced the role of "anthropologist as critic" in this book, I in no way mean to condemn the efforts or malign their good intentions. I also would like to thank Lucia, Aura, Maria Eufemia, and Apolonia for their company during the weeks of door-to-door interviewing, which was frequently challenging. Maria Elena, Josefina, and Isabel all made a great effort to transcribe my recordings. I would like to thank all of the citizens of Santa Cruz, who opened their doors to me and who took care of me when the rest of my family was gone. Finally, I would like to thank the men and women of the Seventh Health District and greater Sololá who gave their time to help with this project.

The initial drafts of this book were made possible by generous funding from the Department of Anthropology, the Institute for Research on Women and Gender, and Rackham Graduate School, all at the University of Michigan. The Department of Health Behavior and Health Education at the University of North Carolina gave me a home for two years, where I was allowed to let my ideas percolate. Time, space, and financial support to revise and re-revise have been provided by the Faculty of Health Sciences at Simon Fraser University.

Several colleagues read earlier drafts of chapters or parts of chapters. I would like to thank Sallie Han, Eric Stein, Elizabeth Roberts, Doug Rogers, and Genese Sodikoff, as well as the Community of Scholars and the Adoption, Infertility, and Gender group, both at the Institute for Research on Women and Gender. Michael Hathaway has been particularly wonderful in helping me clarify my argument. I have tried to incorporate his important insights. Kim Clum deserves special recognition for hashing out many of the raw ideas that undergirded both my research and my writing. She, Bianet Castellaños, and Veronica Benet-Martinez all deserve a word of thanks for visiting me in the field and conversing with me while the topics were still fresh. My fellow Cosmic Lovers have helped enormously and I appreciate their company, encouragement, and willingness to visit me wherever I happen to be at the moment. I particularly appreciate Cristin Colbert's input into the second draft of the manuscript.

There are two people without whom this book would never have come into existence. The first is Jessa Leinaweaver. She encouraged me in the initial drafts of the chapters, spending a lot of time just talking to me about my thoughts and experiences and helping me shape them. Knowing that I had an actual audience for my drafts gave me the impetus to produce something. She has not only read every word in this book, but has read many of the chapters several times. I'm glad that I took up this project if only because it has given me a chance to build my relationship with her.

The second person to whom I owe this book is my academic fairy godmother, Marcia Inhorn. Without Marcia I might never have published one word. It was she that read and reread my work and showed me how to choose an article to publish, sent me a model cover letter, encouraged me when at first I didn't succeed and helped me respond to the reviewers' critiques so that eventually I did. Only by doing those first few articles have I felt confident enough to take on a book project. Before Marcia I had no role model of what I could be when I grew up. I feel fortunate to know such an insightful, compassionate, hard-working, and productive academic who has become such a supportive friend.

Finally, I would like to thank all of my family members for coming to Guatemala to be with me. I am grateful to my husband, Pablo Nepomnaschy, for having the forethought to choose the same field-site. He was the perfect all-around companion for the field. I also appreciate his trips and support when I had to stay in Guatemala without him. As this project has matured with me I have become more indebted to him and my two children, Lucas and Sebastian. I certainly would not have had the strength to walk to my office, sit alone, and face many of the truly depressing aspects of this book were it not for them. Knowing that at the end of the day I would return home to be met with joy and happiness allowed me to fully engage my experience in Guatemala.

I will always be indebted to the people whose intimate stories are told in these pages.

Prologue

THE STORY OF ROSARIO

O n a January morning in 2003 in the village of Santa Cruz La Laguna, Guatemala, Julio came to my house, overheated and out of breath. There was, he said, a "small" problem. His sister-in-law, Rosario, had just given birth to a baby boy, after which she had passed out. She was still unconscious.

I had known Rosario for several years, and was very fond of her, as well as impressed by her ambition and intelligence. Rosario came from one of the most economically prosperous households in the village, and was one of the few young women to graduate from high school. She wanted to continue studying and become a professional—perhaps the first female professional in Santa Cruz. I'd met her when she and her best friend, though barely in their twenties, ran my husband's laboratory.[1] In no time they were processing hundreds of urine and saliva samples a week and had mastered Microsoft Excel. She was well-loved and respected by many in the village.

Rosario had a sporadic relationship with her childhood sweetheart, Marcel. He came from a well-educated family and also had aspirations to be a professional, but in the last few years he had started to drink. Drinking she could handle, but a drunk she could not. In a typical pattern they would be happy together until he lost control of his drinking, after which she would break up with him and he would renounce alcohol forever and beg her to come back. They finally committed to remain together as a couple and she became pregnant. Marcel had built them a house rather high up on the side of the mountain where the town of Santa Cruz perched, and each morning she walked down with him on his way to work and spent the day with her mother. About four months before her brother-in-law Julio showed up at my door, I had visited Rosario in her new home. She seemed very happy. She said that though she and Marcel still had their problems, she hoped that she could learn to stop getting so angry at him, and that he could learn how to stop drinking. All in all, she felt that she had made the right choice and was thrilled to be expecting a baby. As her pregnancy progressed it became more difficult for her to walk up and down the steep hill, and eventually the couple decided to move in with Marcel's parents until the baby was born. His parents lived in the center of town and a small door in the wall of their compound opened onto the courtyard of Rosario's parents' house, so it was very convenient for her.

Though Rosario went to prenatal appointments and her baby seemed fine, her pregnancy was not without incident. Since I had known her she had suffered from chronic anemia. She also had shortness of breath and was underweight. She developed a urinary tract infection (UTI) early in the pregnancy, which she had treated at the doctor. Doña Gladys, the retired nurse who lived in the village, strongly believed Rosario needed to deliver in the hospital, because her anemia put her at risk for complication. She had visited Rosario several times and also told Rosario's in-laws her conviction that Rosario should give birth at the hospital. But in Santa Cruz women and their families almost exclusively preferred homebirth, and it was quite uncommon for a woman to deliver in the hospital. About a month before she was due her UTI returned and she had a fever for a week. I urged her to go to the doctor and treat the infection. She said that her husband could not get time off work and didn't want her to go alone. We arranged that I would accompany her there the next Friday, but she did not come to the appointment. I talked to her husband over the weekend, and said that I would wait again for her on Monday, but again, she never appeared. About two weeks before the baby was born my husband and I visited Rosario and Marcel. By this time I was a year and a half into my research on the high rates of maternal mortality among indigenous women, and I understood how important it was socially for Rosario to deliver her first baby successfully at her in-laws'. I was inclined, therefore, to let her and her family weigh the costs and benefits. Like the nurse, however, my husband was convinced that Rosario needed to have the baby in the hospital because of her now chronic anemia and chronic UTI. He talked to Rosario and Marcel about it, and Marcel said that they would consider it.

With Julio's arrival at my house, it was obvious that Rosario and her family had agreed that a homebirth at her in-laws' would be best. Julio asked if I could come back with him to the house. I went to my bedroom for money and a phone card, and when I returned to the kitchen, Julio was gone. I grabbed the midwifery manual, *Where Women Have No Doctor*, and found Julio's brother Silvio waiting for me outside. We quickly went up the hill to the house of Rosario's in-laws. Wailing came from the room where Rosario and her husband Marcel had been living for the last months. The room was very dark, and the small windows were covered with cloth. There was a loud din from people talking and praying. Someone on the bed rocked Rosario on his lap, which initially made her appear conscious. An elder from the Charismatic Church knelt as he read from the Bible. Julio told me to go to Rosario. She was unconscious.

The nurse was not at the health post, and Doña Gladys, the retired nurse who lived nearby, wasn't at home either. To Julio's disappointment I had no IV solution, nor did I have any idea how to insert an IV had we had one. I asked if she had swelled up right before the birth and he said that she had not. The midwife and Rosario's mother-in-law said that neither had she lost a lot of blood during the birth. I tried to take her pulse but I couldn't tell if the very faint heartbeat was hers or my own. Fearing that she was dead, but hoping there might still be some way to save her, I said that I thought that we should go to the hospital.

The midwife said that she had seen this before and a little IV solution would bring her back to life. Rosario's mother concurred. A debate ensued about getting her an IV versus taking her to the hospital. Her brother and many of her male in-laws wanted to take her to the hospital. I suggested that even if all she needed was a little IV solution, at the hospital they could also diagnose her and prevent any recurrence. Julio had me confirm several times that I thought she should go to the hospital. He knew that I had been working there as part of my research, and so he asked me if my knowing people in the hospital would cause them to attend to Rosario quickly. I replied that I thought that it would. He clearly hoped my suggestions would help galvanize his position among his family members.

It was determined that Marcel, Rosario's mother, the midwife, and I would accompany her to the hospital. The debate then switched to how we would get her there. This was no small concern, as Santa Cruz is accessible by foot and water, but had no road connecting it to the rest of the country. The midwife and several other women bun-

dled Rosario in blankets and shawls, making sure to cover her face.
I knew from having accompanied others to the hospital that people
felt very strongly about protecting the sick from both drafts and on-
lookers. Marcel frantically ran ahead to the police station to call the
firemen, whose responsibility it was to ferry patients between the
dock and the hospital. He alerted them that we were coming and
they said that they would meet us with their truck when we arrived
at the dock in Panajachel.

The family carried Rosario out to the only car in town, a pick-up
truck, to help us quickly traverse the distances between the village
and the dock. Silvio got in the back and heaved her body on top of
himself. Rosario's mother, Doña Inés, sat in front while the rest of us
sat in back with Rosario. At the last minute the midwife declined to
go. As usual, children chased the car as we drove out of the village.
Marcel jumped in when we passed the police station. Halfway down
the hill he called the firemen again from his cell phone, telling them
that we would be there shortly.

When we arrived at the dock Rosario's father shouted to his
nephew to bring the boat over. Our transport would be provided
by a *lancha*—a passenger boat that taxied people back and forth between villages on the lake. Each lancha had four benches that had
been installed and most had a small fiberglass roof that was positioned over the benches. An approaching boat pulled into the only
open slip. Everyone yelled at the driver to move, but he said his
passengers would soon disembark. The boat driver occupying the
second slip moved so that the boat for Rosario could dock, and she
was carried down to the boat by some of the men. While lowering
her onto the deck they dropped her by accident into the hull.

For the five minute trip to the next dock Rosario lay in Silvio's
arms while the church elder again knelt and prayed. I showed Julio
how to take her pulse, and he held onto her wrist tightly as he prayed.
Various family members shouted to Marcel that Rosario needed air,
so he uncovered her face. They then instructed him to fan her with
a piece of cloth. He searched madly for something to use and eventually took off his shirt and waved it in her face.

No ambulance awaited us at the next dock, so Marcel called again
to notify them of our arrival. Another boat was parked in the only
slot, and again members of our party shouted at the driver to move it
quickly. Soon we docked, and the congregation elder and I went up
to the road to find the ambulance. After it arrived we took the stretcher down to the dock. A few of the men put Rosario on the stretcher
and carried her to the ambulance. Marcel and Julio got in with her,

with Silvio slipping in at the last minute, as the driver had said only two others were allowed in back. Doña Inés and I rode up front.

In the emergency room we encountered two healthcare professionals: a male doctor and a female nurse, both dressed in blue scrubs. The doctor, who was across the room, yelled for us to tell him what had happened to her. The ambulance driver replied that Rosario had lost consciousness. The doctor asked if she had fallen. Someone in the family said she had not fallen, but rather she had lost consciousness while giving birth. I then explained that she had delivered the baby and the placenta and then passed out at around 11:00 AM that morning. According to my watch, it was now 12:15 PM.

The doctor opened up her skirt so that she was naked from the waist down. He bent her knees and placed the soles of her feet together so that her legs bowed, and lowered his head a little to look at her vagina. Then he pressed on her bladder, which caused urine to trickle out. Everyone in her family remained still, their faces utterly impassive.

The doctor instructed the nurse to insert an IV and then stated that only one person could remain with the patient. He closed the curtain around her bed and returned to his desk. Since bringing Rosario to the hospital Silvio had been sitting behind her to hold her upright, and at this point Marcel switched places with him. It was important to her in-laws that she remain upright.

Despite the doctor's directive I stayed with Marcel. The nurse, in latex gloves, asked us to remove Rosario's sweater. Once some of her clothing was off the nurse noticed the large cloth belt that the midwife had tied around Rosario's ribs, which she also instructed us to remove. She and I tried to untie it but it was knotted too tightly. I attempted to saw it apart with Marcel's knife. Finally the nurse used scissors to sever the belt, and we unwrapped it.

The doctor returned with his stethoscope and pen light. He tried to find a pulse on the inside of Rosario's elbow, then on her chest, and finally on the side of her neck. The nurse was unable to find a vein for the IV. The doctor held open her eyelids and shined his pen light into her eyes. I realized then that she was really dead. Marcel shifted her, attempting to get her in a better position. Her jet black hair, which was now, as always, so shiny, thick, and meticulously braided, dropped down behind her. Marcel kissed her and murmured to her. He believed that she was still alive. The nurse said that she couldn't find a vein, and the doctor told her, "*Esta ya esta muerta*" [This one is already dead]. And that was how we got the news. It seemed to be in that moment, really, that she died. Marcel and I raised our hands, turned away, covered our faces and began to sob. The doctor and nurse asked us to leave because we were making a scene. I handed Marcel back his knife and we left the ER.

When we walked into the waiting area, we saw that all of Rosario's relatives had arrived. I reported to them that the doctor said that she had died. As I had no information about what had caused her death, I returned to Rosario's bed and found that the doctor was still with her in the ER. He said hemorrhage was the cause of death. I said that I had specifically asked the midwife about bleeding, and that everyone present at the birth had agreed that Rosario had not lost a lot of blood. He told me to look at the color of her gums and lips, which were a whitish-gray. They were that color, he said, because she had lost all of her blood and didn't have any left.

Outside, among her family, a heated conversation resumed about how Rosario just needed an IV. Marcel returned to the ER and begged them to try to insert the IV. The doctor said that it wouldn't do any good, because she was already dead. I asked the doctor to explain why an IV wouldn't do any good now, but he wouldn't. Her family was enraged that the doctor wouldn't give her an IV and was complaining that the hospital refused to treat her. The church elder went to speak with the doctor and again asked him to put in the IV. Again the doctor refused.

I returned to the ER and asked what would happen next. The doctor responded that since she had died before her arrival there, they had sent the body to the morgue, where the pathologist would do an autopsy. I asked how long that would take and he said that he couldn't say. When pressed he asked someone else in the ER, who said that the people in the funeral parlor across the street were more familiar with the process and would be able to tell us when we could get the body back.

When I returned again to the waiting area, everyone was sobbing. Doña Inés began to beat and scream at Marcel. She said that it was all his fault, that all he ever did was hurt Rosario and bring her pain. Rosario was gone because of him, and also because of him we were here in the hospital. Marcel just stood there while Doña Ines berated him. Finally his family pulled him away.

Gradually the family dispersed. Some went to the morgue to be with the body, while others went to the funeral parlor. I remained outside the emergency room, because I thought I might be of use there, and also because I was uncertain what else to do. My watch still said 12:15 PM. In fact my watch had stopped and it was really 1:20 PM. I estimated that we had arrived at the hospital at about

12:45 PM. Julio came back to find me and told me that an official from the Ministry of Health would need to certify that Rosario's death was natural and not a murder, after which the autopsy would be waived. Julio wanted me to talk to the official, but I worried my presence might lead the official to try for a larger bribe. Also foreigners had a reputation for being sticklers for rules, so the official might not be willing to "work it out"—that is, take a bribe at all—if I was there. I suggested that Julio first try to negotiate, and contact me if he ran into trouble.

Three women from other Kaqchikel lake villages were in the waiting area outside the ER. They had heard that a woman from Santa Cruz, which was a neighboring Kaqchikel village, had just arrived and died, and they were discussing the case. The woman from San Jorge said that she had met Rosario, and that she was a wonderful person. The woman from Santa Catarina thought that it was terrible that Rosario was already dead and they were still going to "operate" on her, referring to the autopsy. The other two agreed. The woman from San Jorge said that if we had bribed the doctor, he would have claimed she arrived alive and died in the hospital. That way, we could have taken the body home quickly.

After the women dispersed I still remained waiting outside the ER. The Ministry of Health official came, but Julio was unsuccessful in having the autopsy canceled. The official had called the pathologist, who was in Guatemala City and would have to travel three hours to Sololá to perform the autopsy.

I accompanied Julio back to the morgue, where all of Rosario's in-laws were sitting against the wall, and the woman from San Jorge was attempting to console Doña Inés. A policeman came up with a notebook and asked for the name of the midwife. Marcel looked at him and said, "The truth is I don't know what to tell you." He asked the others what her name was and they suggested Maria, with the surname of either Saloj or Chumil or something along those lines, but they couldn't be sure. I knew that they were making up these guesses and were actually quite certain of the midwife's name, but I kept silent. Rosario's younger brother said there was no reason to stay since the pathologist would not be there before 5:00 PM. Doña Inés wanted to leave, and I accompanied all of Rosario's family members as we left the hospital. Her son had a taxi waiting, which delivered us to the dock where we took the boat back to Santa Cruz.

Late that night the boat carrying Rosario's body arrived in Santa Cruz. The family had borrowed a welded steel frame from the church to carry the coffin up to the village. Because of the geography of

Santa Cruz, where the village was embedded in a steep mountain side, driving a coffin from the dock to the house and then to the cemetery was not possible. Rather, young men volunteered to carry the coffin, using the frame, up to the town. At least a hundred people, including potential pall bearers, were waiting for Rosario's return. The family unloaded the coffin, put it on the frame, and everyone walked behind it in a procession to Marcel's parents' house. The casket was placed in the room where, that morning, she had given birth, and died. The funeral was scheduled for 2:00 PM the next day.

Four days after Rosario's death, I went to the headquarters of the Ministry of Health in Sololá (the location of the hospital) and asked the director for the results of the autopsy. I relayed how the emergency room doctor had told me that the cause of death was hemorrhage, but I hadn't seen any blood either on the sheets of the bed, the bedspread, or her clothes. I speculated that her family might have changed the sheets before I had arrived, which the director thought was probably the case. The pathologist at the morgue said that she died from *atonia uterina* [uterine atony], meaning that her uterus never contracted after the birth, causing her to continue to bleed until she went into hypovolemic shock and eventually died.

The official interpretation of Rosario's death, however, was radically different from how her death was explained in the village. Everyone there was certain that she had died of a heart attack. Rosario was known in the village for having a weak heart—she was frequently short of breath—and most people found it reasonable that her heart just couldn't take the strain of childbirth. The nurse, for a verbal autopsy, separately interviewed her husband and the midwife. Each emphasized the fact that one second she was fine, asking for tea, and the next second she was unconscious. The quickness and extremity of the change convinced them that she had had a heart attack. When the nurse asked about blood, they each denied that any blood had been present after the birth. She then asked if anyone had changed the sheets after the birth and they each denied that such had occurred.

Though most everyone in Santa Cruz agreed that Rosario had died of a heart attack, the explanations of what caused the heart attack varied. Some believed her weak heart had simply given out during the birth, while others felt that her heart attack was provoked by witchcraft directed at the midwife. The midwife who delivered Rosario's baby had recently almost lost two other patients, and Rosario's death seemed too much to be a coincidence.

Rosario's family, on the other hand, was certain that it was Marcel's fault for rousing the jealousy of a scorned woman. They said that Marcel, before marrying Rosario, had fathered babies with other women and then denied paternity. One of these women had taken her revenge by bewitching Rosario. Rosario's parents threatened to go to a powerful shaman in another village who would be able to tell them who had killed their daughter. They were certain that the guilt would fall on Marcel, turning him into an outcast. However, although much bitterness and blame followed Rosario's death, her parents never went to the shaman.

In her short life, Rosario left behind a son, named in her honor. Seeing this beautiful boy, who has the same birthmarks as his mother, is always bittersweet for me.

Introduction

THE SPECTER OF DEATH

This book is about maternal mortality, or pregnancy-related death, and its impact. My focus is to explore some consequences of how the global community has tried to prevent these deaths from happening. I argue that the global campaign to decrease maternal mortality has actually created barriers to reducing deaths and also threatens to make some of the very communities that it is designed to help even more vulnerable.

In the more than twenty years that pregnancy-related death has been on the international agenda, our understanding of it has become overly circumscribed. Essentially, maternal mortality has been reduced to a medical problem where lack of access to skilled biomedical providers dominates the agenda for making pregnancy safer. The evaluation of our effort has involved ever increasing surveillance of maternal mortality rates and biomedical skills relating to emergency obstetrics. An unspoken effect of reducing maternal mortality to a medical problem is that life and death become the *only* outcomes by which pregnancy and birth are understood. The specter of death looms large and limits our full exploration of either our attempts to curb maternal mortality, or the phenomenon itself.

Certainly women's survival during childbirth is the ultimate measure of success of our efforts. Yet using pregnancy outcomes and biomedical attendance at birth as the primary feedback on global efforts to make pregnancy safer is misguided. First, as I discuss in chapter 3, our measures of maternal deaths are woefully poor indicators of the effects of an intervention. Second, we neglect to monitor the potential impacts of the international Safe Motherhood campaign

as a global blueprint for how to mobilize monetary and human resources, and script local daily interactions concerning pregnancy
and birth worldwide. We know that life and death are not the only
outcomes that are important to women or their families in relation
to pregnancy and birth. The forced biomedicalization of birth and
the abuses that poor women like Rosario suffer at the hands of biomedical practitioners during this vulnerable and liminal period are
central to women's concerns.[1] Third, we neglect the myriad rich and
important other sources of data that might help us mitigate some of
these deaths.

In other words, the global campaign to decrease maternal mortality has incredible potential to disrupt women's daily lives, yet little
effort has been made to evaluate any dimension of this effort other
than its ability to prevent death. The more this campaign has focused
on the biomedical management of pregnancy and birth, the more it
has advocated standardizing the everyday practices related to the
control of these events around the world. But the narrow rhetorical
space in which this campaign has taken place has concentrated on
international agents engaged in a battle against obstetric pathology,
and the question of what actually happens when health systems and
development agents try to lower maternal mortality has been invisible. Denise Roth Allen (2002) and Craig R. Janes and Oyuntsetseg
Chuluundorj (2004) have recently demonstrated how to move forward by confronting Safe Motherhood as more than a transparent
attempt to save the lives of women. My book continues this effort by
examining the actual effects of the global campaign and pushing to
broaden the conversation about maternal mortality and its causes.

Interrupting a Global Campaign
to Help Make Birth Safer

An obvious reason this ethnography is important is to help us better
understand why decreasing maternal mortality around the globe is
so difficult, but this case study is also critical to helping each of us
understand globalization and global citizenship. From my perspective, ethnography has a vital role to play not necessarily in defining
"globalization," but rather in interrupting its narrative of inevitable
western dominance that exculpates those of us living in the developed world from seeing, acting on, or challenging injustice. Examining a global health project can help each of us, as scholars, teachers,
and students, realize what is at stake when we fail to question or

examine attempts to—in John F. Kennedy's terms—"help them help themselves."

So I start with the claim that an ethnography of Safe Motherhood can help us learn about globalization.[2] In its most dominant version, globalization theory accounts for an inevitable, global transformation where a world rich in variety gets squeezed through a bottleneck to produce a more uniform, homogenous world.[3] As Jan Nederveen Pieterse (1995:45) summarizes popular takes on the process of globalization, "the world is becoming more uniform and standardized through a technological, commercial and cultural synchronization emanating from the West." Arjun Appadurai (1990:295) emphasizes the connection between a world looking more "western" and the uniform spread of global capitalism when he claims that globalization frequently contains "an argument about 'commoditization.'"

I am suspicious of globalization theory because it smacks of being a "stor[y] we tell ourselves about ourselves" (Geertz 1973:8). The primary "we" who tell the story of globalization are those who live in the global North. And the storyline itself can be roughly translated into "everyone wants to be (or is inevitably becoming) more like us." Looked at from this perspective, globalization theory sounds remarkably like what Gananath Obeyesekere (1992) refers to as "European myth-making."

Is it true that everyone wants to be like the global North? Is that really where the world is going? Is it inevitable? Anthropologists who have written before me have persuasively provided a counter-discourse to what Kalman Applbaum (2000:258) aptly describes as the "cheerful version" of an inevitable westernized world. When we look at what happens on the ground we can see that globalization is not a steam roller and people around the world are not passive recipients. Instead of traveling unimpeded into a "cultural void," the processes of globalization are significantly shaped by a diversity of "local" practices and beliefs (Inhorn 2003).[4] Globalization doesn't just happen; rather, individuals in diverse settings from all over the world are implicated in accommodating, negotiating, or resisting change.[5] Empirical accounts have taught us that globalization does not have any one desired effect. Anna Lowenhaupt Tsing (2005) argues that her own empirical accounts contain the details necessary to "fragment" what may at first appear to be a "well-oiled machine," thereby subverting the idea of "smooth global integration."[6] Finally, anthropologists such as Karen Ho (2005:86) have cautioned us to consider globalization "not simply a[s] fact, but a hope, a strategy, and a triumphalist ideology."[7]

My own attempt to answer questions about inevitable western-
ization focuses on the translation (Pigg 2001) of a global health campaign in a particular place at a particular historical moment. I want
to show how the meanings of the global campaign to lower maternal mortality are mediated by the health workers in Sololá whose
job it is to implement global policies. Importantly, what this global
campaign comes to represent in Sololá is surely not what was intended in the conference rooms in Geneva or New York, where such
policies are hammered out. Rather, front-line health workers interpreted the tools and technologies of the global fight against maternal
mortality to fit locally familiar narratives. Health workers in Sololá
inextricably linked the fight against maternal mortality with efforts
to forge national unity in the chaotic and violent aftermath of an
even more vicious civil war. The global campaign piggybacked on a
narrative of national progress and modernization that was used to
justify rooting out "backwardness" that endangered this progress.
For health workers, the global campaign against maternal mortality
provided an objective, neutral framework to cloak their own prejudice toward certain types of difference. For example, it problema-
tized obstetric practices preferred by many poor, indigenous Maya,
such as birthing at home with a traditional midwife instead of with a
biomedical provider in the hospital. It also attempted to subtly erode
these practices and the understandings of the world that organized
them.

This account of attempts to decrease maternal mortality inter-
rupts the "story" of globalization and the moral cover that it provides
for processes that should, in fact, be questioned. When globalization
is allowed to remain a metaphorical phone booth that converts all
who enter it into Westerners, we lose sight of our own collusion
in the process. Only by recognizing that the medication that I buy
or the vote that I cast can be intimately connected to exploitation,
structural violence, empowerment, and "well-being" on the other
side of the globe, can I consciously participate in a construction of
the global. Yet I consider the imperative of interrupting what Frederick Cooper (2001) refers to as the global "juggernaut," specifically
tied to my responsibilities as a teacher. David L. Blaney (2002) in-
sists that engaging students in a valuable conversation about the
global depends on problematizing their own social privilege, and not
allowing them to take it for granted.[8] Challenging the inevitabilities
of the global conversion to the West is one means of drawing us all
into a conversation that recognizes the complexities and specificities
of the processes we refer to as globalization.

Biosocial Subjectivities: The Meaning of Making Babies

I contend that one of the significant consequences of the global Safe Motherhood campaign has been to unintentionally encourage a shift in subjectivity among Kaqchikel Maya villagers with whom I lived in Guatemala. While *subjectivity* is a term that has a certain "openness of ... meaning today" (Biehl, Good, and Kleinman 2007:15), I simply use it to refer to someone's own understanding of his or her place in the world. Subjectivity is about an individual's internal processes, dispositions, or understandings, as opposed to other people's judgments or attributions about an individual.

Highlighting the biosocial nature of subjectivities helps us understand how global Safe Motherhood might provoke a subjective shift. I use the term *biosocial subjectivities* to emphasize that our own understandings of our place in the world are necessarily mediated by and reflective of our biological processes. In other words, biosocial subjectivity draws our attention to the necessary symmetry between our bodily experiences and how we understand ourselves. Perhaps this relationship has been most evocatively drawn out in bird's-eye-view studies of gender that show how treatments of bodies (Boddy 1989) and understandings of bodies (Delaney 1991; Kaspin 1996) map so well onto more holistic renderings of self and society. My emphasis on biological processes and bodily experiences intentionally shifts our attention away from the body as an object per se and toward an exploration of biological processes and actions.[9]

I use *biosocial* as it is used in a number of disciplines, including anthropology, to signal that a particular phenomenon must be analyzed with reference to both the biological and social. On a lexical level, biosocial shares much with Paul Rabinow's (1996:99) concept of biosociality, which inverts the nature/culture distinction by revealing scientific systems as cultural systems, and thereby recognizing that culture is how we come to know about the world. In my larger analysis, I certainly argue that the global Safe Motherhood campaign is dependent on cultural understandings of birth and birthing-related problems rather than any "natural" understandings that it might claim. Nevertheless, I do not carry Rabinow's thought experiment anywhere near its logical conclusion. Semantically, no overlap is intended here between my use of biosocial and biosociality, and metaphysically my analysis differs from his. By invoking biosocial, I intend to suggest that it is analytically productive to consider the biological and social as two different domains that mutually constitute our world. My analysis assumes that the two are intertwined, but leaves aside questions of whether or not one is dominant over or constitutive of the other.

Perhaps Brigitte Jordan (1978:1) has most productively used the idea of biosocial in her groundbreaking ethnography to show that pregnancy and birth across the globe must be understood as "biosocial event[s] [that] recognize at the same time the universal biological function and the culture-specific social matrix within which human biology is embedded." It is important to read Jordan's statement in relation to the temporal context in which it was written. For the purposes of using it today, I would gloss references to "universal biological function" as referring to the propensity of women across the world to get pregnant and give birth. We certainly understand that not all women can (Inhorn and Balen 2002) or do birth and that what seems to be universally biological can be as heterogeneous as it assumed to be homogenous (Lock 1993). Nevertheless, by employing a biosocial framework, Jordan was able to instantiate that birth could not be considered as a solely physiological process, but demands a conjoined cultural analysis. The legacy of her insight has organized much subsequent work on birth and reproduction, including my own.

While Jordan employed a biosocial framework to highlight the social and the cultural, my intention in employing the term *biosocial subjectivity* is to emphasize the importance of understanding the relationship between subjectivities and biological processes.[10] Michel Foucault (1978) has drawn our attention the great potential of the biological domain to mediate understandings of self through his concept of biopower. Many of the mechanisms that the State uses to consolidate power over its citizens directly involve propagating discourses about biological processes. His analysis reveals how central our experience and understandings of our own biological processes are to subject-making. By controlling discourses around biological processes the State is able to produce self-disciplining subjects that do not threaten State power. In sum, influencing discourse around biological processes is a mechanism that the State uses to produce particular subjectivities that it is able to subjugate.

I am following Foucault's lead in drawing attention to the privileged position that biological processes hold in subject-making, and I argue that pregnancy and birth are some of the most important sites for shaping our subjectivity. As social beings, humans are seeped in contexts of culture, and ideas of continuity and reproduction (as well as disruption) of culture are central to society. Yet cultures cannot be produced or reproduced without new members. The processes through which new members are procured are myriad (e.g., marriage, adoption, conversion, etc.), but making new members from one's own body holds a particularly important place. Pregnancy and birth are the physiological processes that create the next generation. They are, accordingly, particularly charged locations from which to define and reproduce the social world. Pregnancy and birth should then serve as comparatively robust sites from which to understand biosocial subjectivities.

Yet, unlike Foucault, my exploration of biosocial subjectivities is not focused on the link between discourses around pregnancy and birth and State (or global Safe Motherhood) power. While this ethnography certainly could be read as a story about State-produced shifts in subjectivities that increase its own power over the indigenous population, I don't find such an orientation analytically productive. That story reads far too much like our current stories about globalization where the outcome—increase of State power and loss of subject autonomy—is foretold. By shifting our analytical lens we can instead focus on parts of this research that remain obscured: What are the empirical ways that pregnancy and birth are linked to wider social life that make them important subject-forming locations? What does this mean, in particular, for public health interventions aimed at those sites? How has global Safe Motherhood worked to alter subjectivities by changing everyday events surrounding these important biological processes? What tangible consequences might such interventions in birth have for communities, such as those in Sololá?

In this ethnography, I argue that global Safe Motherhood's cultural understanding of pregnancy and birth as primarily physiological processes have worked in Guatemala to promote autonomous, as opposed to mutually constituted or connective subjectivities. The cultural understanding of pregnancy and birth are well highlighted by Rosario's birth story. In the version of her story favored by the global campaign, and demonstrated by the health system in Sololá, Rosario's anemia contributed to an acute post-partum hemorrhage. The description of what went wrong was essentially derived from her autopsy, and focused exclusively on the internal factors that caused her difficulties (e.g., failure of her uterus to contract). While the former version of the story may appear to a biomedically oriented reader as neutral, medical anthropologists have persuasively demonstrated that even descriptive work, such as mapping chromosomes (Rapp 1999) or describing reproduction (Martin 1992), is framed culturally. Perhaps most helpfully, Davis-Floyd (1992) deconstructed hospital birthing events in the US to show how obstetric protocol could be just as much about culture as it was about medicine.

Perhaps the particular, cultural orientation of the Safe Motherhood campaign is more obvious when it is juxtaposed to the version of events that dominated Rosario's village. In this version, a malevolent person induced Rosario to suffer a heart attack with the aid of a witch. Both birth and birthing problems were understood through reference to social relationships in contrast to physiological ones. Village gossip pegged the root of her birthing trouble externally, on a spurned woman—not on the internal physiological mechanism that this woman might have employed to take revenge, i.e., the heart attack. In sum, both models prioritize a certain way of understanding birth. The emphasis on the social aspects of birth prioritized in Rosario's village can be critically applied to the global campaign to reveal how the health system ignores the potential of birth as a site to make meaning about social relationships. What might such a disruption of opportunity to make meaning imply? Is it important, and if so, how?

As Rosario's difficult birth story illustrates, the potential involvement of extensive kin make pregnancy and birth events special locations to (re)define social relationships—particularly kin relations. I follow in the footsteps of anthropologists who have found it instructive to attend to the definitions of kin terms such as "husband" or "daughter" as they are defined processually, rather than focusing on how they are determined by blood.[11] Kaqchikel pregnancy and homebirths are robust sites for studying how relationships are performed, as each can require the participation of husbands, parents, in-laws, grandparents, aunts, uncles, and sometimes even other children. For example, when a husband physically supports his wife so that she can maintain a squatting position during labor, what it means to be a husband or a wife is both enacted and reinstantiated.

The involvement described above where a number of kin participate in the typical homebirth simultaneously reflects and reinstantiates an understanding of one's place in the world as related to and constituted by others. In other words, the homebirth encourages a relational subjectivity. It reinforces the idea that, in Marilyn Strathern's (1988:13) words, "persons are frequently constructed as the ... composite site of relationships that produced them."[12] The individual ceases to have any discrete meaning beyond those relationships. In her provocative work on connectivity in brother-sister relationships, Suad Joseph (1994:55) gives us a glimpse of the everyday actions that illustrate how "connective persons ... require the involvement of others in shaping their emotions, desires, attitudes and identities." She details interactions between siblings to demonstrate the "processes by which one person comes to see him/herself as part of another,"[13] further helping us delineate what constitutes a relational subjectivity.

Perhaps the easiest way to understand what it means to say that a particular process of birth reinstantiates subjectivity is to consider the converse: another birth process (e.g., hospital birth) can promote an understanding of individuals as autonomous. Just looking at a snapshot to compare the two events can help us with this conceptualization (see Illustration 1 and Illustration 2).

Illustration 1 depicts a hospital birth in the United States. Illustration 2 is a painting of a homebirth in a Mayan community in Sololá. Regardless of whether or not these illustrations are typical, overlaying a kinship diagram onto these two birthing events certainly helps us understand the relationship between the experience of a biological process and one's understanding of self. While the physiological details of each birth might have significant overlap, the social matrix in which the birthing event is located is profoundly different. One event prioritizes kin connections. In the other, individuals are disconnected.

I argue that the Safe Motherhood campaign encourages a shift in subjectivity by organizing everyday events around birth to em-

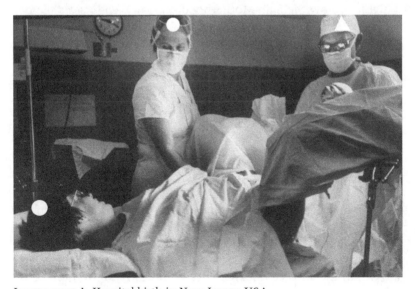

ILLUSTRATION 1. Hospital birth in New Jersey, USA

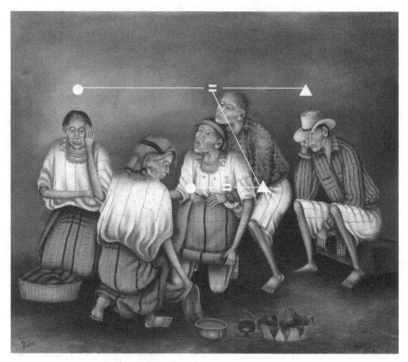

ILLUSTRATION 2. Homebirth in Atitlan, Guatemala

phasize birth as a physiological process. In the subsequent chapters I highlight how the Safe Motherhood campaign endorses a biologization of birth. We can easily see this biologization in the definition of the causes of maternal mortality, the organization of resources around skilled attendance, and the inevitable push for more hospital births. Yet, as I argue, shifting Kaqchikel village births from home to hospital necessarily engenders a shift in how both the woman who gives birth and her kin who attend a birth understand their places in the world.

Subjectivity and Globalization

Scholars writing about subjectivity and globalization have used two different lines of inquiry to understand transformations associated with the global. The first approach concentrates on trying to understand how transformations in subjectivities happen. The second attends to the subjective experience of globalization more broadly.

Of course the two lines of inquiry are not mutually exclusive, and I have tried to connect what is happening in Sololá to both.

Despite the fact that globalization is arguably not the homogenous, all-powerful transformative process that some might assume, invoking globalization writ-large still opens a discussion about transformations. How do global processes transform subjectivities? Foucault has contributed generously to this discussion. One of his primary insights has been to illustrate how subjectivities are the products of particular historical moments and are intricately bound to the cultures and institutions in conjunction with which they are formed (1978, 1983). Foucault's insight helps us view subjectivities as part of a specific (social ecological) system. Subjectivities are, therefore, variable across both time and space. Foucault also emphasizes subjectivities' dependence on the larger macro elements of the system for their own definition. He deftly sketches out the terms of this dependence by attending to the intertwining of knowledge and power to produce subjects. His works on prisons, clinics, madhouses, and other institutions help show how experts' beliefs and verbal articulations, or discourses, shape society members' own understandings. The basis of a discourse is not truth, yet these discourses differentiate, for example, sick from well or normal from abnormal. The central point is not just that experts see these divides, but discourses form part of one's own understanding of the world. This produces an effect of self-discipline, where individuals internalize and uphold understandings of the world promulgated by discourses.

Foucault's theories help to elucidate the critical impact that ramping up the dissemination of biomedical discourses about pregnancy and birth in Sololá can have on subject formation. As Foucault helps us understand, these causal explanations of birthing difficulties are not divorced from how we understand the world, or our place in the world. Rather, both our subjectivity and our casual explanations of birthing difficulties are developed with respect to the same institutions and fields of discourse. A biomedical model that emphasizes direct causes, or the primarily physiological pathologies that result in death, has been emphasized by global Safe Motherhood and is easily identified in the Ministry of Health's analysis of Rosario's demise. The individual, Rosario, is taken as the unit of analysis. A physiological failure—that is a lack of contraction of her uterus—is identified as the cause of her death. The inability of her uterus to contract at that crucial moment after birth is regarded as random or inexplicable. From this logic stems the idea that the best interventions are those that connect failing individual pregnant or birthing bodies with skilled attendants who will know how to treat hypertensive disorder, hemorrhage, infection, obstructed birth, or an unsafe abortion—the most common pregnancy-related pathologies. On a theoretical level, the ability to globalize these interventions depends on reductionist abstractions of the individual as a discrete physiological system: e.g., whoever you are, wherever you are, a shot of Pitocin should make your uterus cramp. In sum, I argue that the discourses of biomedicine upon which the global interventions to decrease maternal mortality are built, propagate a particular western, autonomous subject.[14]

Foucault's work also indexes a tension concerning the power of states and other larger institutions over the daily lives of individuals. Yet many allege that this is where the limits of his theorizing lie (Sangren 1995; Cooper 1994; Sivaramakrishnan 1995). A rich discussion of agency, or the ability of individuals to influence their own lives, is missing from his writings. While Foucault certainly helps us arrive at a better understanding of the role of power in co-opting knowledge production and generating discourses, he leaves us with an underdeveloped sense of the potency of individuals to create and shape those discourses themselves. In other words, many argue that Foucault's emphasis on power and institutions does not prepare us to understand or predict how people work to transform the world they live in, be it through violent or non-violent social movements, or just individual actions.[15] Scholars who work on agency, such as James C. Scott (1985), describe an individual's ability to transform their world because they possess an original subjectivity that enables them to see the travesty of discourses imposed upon them by institutions such as the State. This original subjectivity enables individuals to exercise their own will and resist (and transform) institutions that would attempt to control them.

While both the "power over" the subject (e.g., Foucault) and the "resistance of" the subject (e.g., Scott) sides of the spectrum have their merit, grounding an analysis on one side or the other can be problematic. Arun Agrawal (2005:170) critiques the one end of the spectrum for a "tendency toward the colonization of the imagination by powerful political beliefs ... and the other [for] the tendency toward durability of a sovereign consciousness founded on the bedrock of individual or class interest." As he points out, subjectivity must be (re)habilitated by finding a middle ground.

Trying to operate in the middle ground certainly buys some flexibility, yet both of these frameworks have particular weaknesses for understanding the relationship between globalization and subjectivity. The "power over" version basically articulates all subjectivities in relation to the same set of historically situated power structures. In my discussion above about interpreting birthing problems I certainly agree that subjectivities are formed in relation to wider social institutions. Yet with respect to globalization, however, is there really a commensurability of a global subject across space? For example, in this analysis, I allege that the autonomous subject is being circulated on the back of Safe Motherhood interventions worldwide. Yet, digging deeper into my own analysis, while I can read the autonomous subject into the journals and literature on Safe Motherhood, in Sololá I could only find it interpreted and shaped by local contexts and actors. This layer of shaping by local actors means that understanding the influence of globalization on subjectivities in multiple locales needs to be more nuanced than simply assuming that one global subjectivity is "colonizing … the imagination" (Agrawal 2005). Furthermore, Foucault has given us little material that we could use to theorize relational subjectivities. Rather, the subject is assumed to be, to some extent, the unit upon which discourses act. Social life is triangulated back to the central discourse. So how do we account for or theorize subjects who triangulate upon each other to understand their place in the world? Finally, I find the presupposition of linearity in relation to subject-making in the "resistance of" versions of subjectivity similarly constraining. The "resistance of" model presupposes a point in time where an obdurate consciousness exists, which at a later time hegemonic, global forces attempt to inscribe. Like the "power over" model, the "resistance of" model imposes a focus on questions concerning the relative dominance of one subjectivity over another, or the origin of subjectivities. In my project, these focuses distract my ability to develop a grounded description of the relationship between subjectivities and globalization.

Alternatively, drawing on models that can accommodate multiple subjectivities could help develop our understanding of the relationship between subjectivities and globalization. Facsimiles of the globally promoted subjects, like the autonomous subject who is the assumed client of global Safe Motherhood campaigns, certainly exist in Santa Cruz. But rather than rolling over and replacing the "authentic" relational subject, these subjectivities coexist. Whether one sees one's place in the world as being defined relationally or autonomously is not a question of either/or, but rather more or less. Like bicultural individuals, context and events prime a person to emphasize one mode of understanding over another (Hong et al. 2000). For example, walking through the city wearing "western" clothes might inspire a different understanding of one's place in the world than assisting one's wife while she gives birth. P. Sean Brotherton's (2008) description of complex subjects simultaneously navigating Cuba's socialists and capitalist-inspired medical systems provides another example of this type of approach. Mikhail Bakhtin's (1981) ideas of how linkages and borrowings that occur during interactions create social meaning provide an alternative "origins story" for subjectivities: temporal linearity is replaced by complex and convoluted constructions of meaning, the origins of which are not only untraceable, but are seemingly less important. The idea that subjectivities are always under construction helps us understand how they could change. Nevertheless, shifts in subjectivity cannot be understood without linking them to shifts of larger institutions.[16]

My approach to helping us understand the relationship between subjectivities and globalization, then, is to provide a detailed ethnography of everyday social interactions. I consider how we understand our own place in the world largely as a collaborative project.[17] Our subjectivities are constructed and reconstructed through daily interactions (Mahmood 2005), and these interactions provide the nexus between how someone understands his or her place in the world, and the everyday events that he or she participates in. By anchoring specific real-time social situations that occur in particular historical moments to wider institutions, such as the Guatemalan State, we are in a position to understand how the larger political-economy serves as a motivator in constructing everyday life. Because of my close attention to everyday interactions, in this ethnography we can only see the global and the State through proxies. These proxies can be, for example, the actions of individuals who imagine the State, or the specific ways that global policies shape daily action. My framework allows for a representation of the real variation in how globalization is operationalized, and a grounded, empirical description of how it might impact or shape subjectivities.

Centering my ethnography in everyday interactions has allowed me to describe the relationship between globalization and subjectivity by attending to the lived experience of those with whom I've worked (Biehl, Good, and Kleinman 2007). Like colonialism, globalization is often a violent process, particularly for the poor and disenfranchised. João Biehl, Byron Good, and Arthur Kleinman (2007) critique academics who study subjectivity and globalization but who gloss over the brutality of the experience in favor of enriching theory. They contend that "[t]heories of subjectivity are too often overstated, obscure, and even dehumanizing. People who are subject to the most profound human experience—suffering massive violence and incomprehensible cruelty, the routine degradation of poverty and despair, the terrors of madness and life-threatening disease, or even facing the impossible dilemmas of providing care, whether surrounded by the highest technologies or near total absence of resources—have too often been transformed into remote abstractions, discursive forms, or subject positions" (13). By attending to the lived experience of indigenous peoples in Sololá, we can also begin to see why questions about subjectivity and globalization are actually far from academic and actually do matter. On a functional level, in an economically impoverished and often violent setting this relational (rather than autonomous) subjectivity can literally form the barrier between life and death. In a State that suffers from a lack of political, legal, and financial resources for poor Maya, a relational subjectivity translates into obligations that frequently provide the only available (albeit flawed) social safety net. In sum, changing birthing practices do matter—these changes can unintentionally transform Maya subjectivities in a way that contributes to weakening the social safety net upon which poor, disenfranchised Maya rely. Ultimately, the global effort to make birth safer may unwittingly generate conditions that jeopardize a population, creating a greater risk than maternal mortality threatens.

Constructing the Field in Sololá, Guatemala

The seeds of this project were sown in 1999 when I had a conversation with the director of the Ministry of Health (MSPAS)[18] in Sololá about the problem of maternal mortality among Mayan women. Based on his suggestion, I returned in August of 2000 and set up shop in Santa Cruz La Laguna. Santa Cruz is a Kaqchikel village on the shore of Lake Atitlan that had about twelve hundred inhabitants at the time of this study. It is the seat of the municipality of Santa Cruz, one of nineteen municipalities that administratively belong to the *departamento* of Sololá. While technically only about seventy-five kilometers from the capital, Guatemala City, Santa Cruz was distinctive for its relative isolation; it could only be accessed by boat or foot. Perhaps because of this "antiquated" arrangement, *Cruceños,* inhabitants of Santa Cruz, have a reputation among other Mayan groups around the lake for being closed, backward, and traditional.

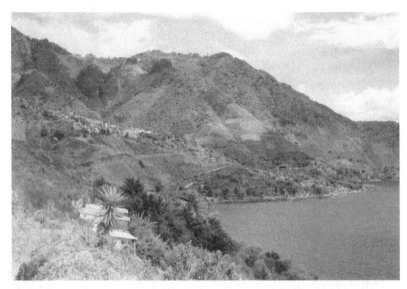

ILLUSTRATION 3. The village of Santa Cruz

I arrived in Santa Cruz fluent in Spanish and English, but I basically spent my first year in the field studying Kaqchikel. My teacher was a man from Santa Cruz, who was more or less my age, fluent in Spanish, and who had graduated from high school. He was one of the few Cruceños who could write Kaqchikel, which was important to me. Over the year that I studied I made a dictionary and created written dialogues about daily aspects of life (such as going to the market, buying tortillas, greeting people on the path, etc.). As my Kaqchikel advanced I would record my teacher telling stories, and then transcribe these stories. Learning the language really dictated the terms of my entrance into Santa Cruz, as I got to hear many more stories and histories of the village, its geographical surroundings, and its inhabitants than normally would have come up in conversation.

While my language-learning activities oriented me to much of day-to-day life, Cruceños were aware that I was there because of my interest in women's reproductive health. The more I became settled, the more I was sought out to deal with those sorts of matters. Women asked me to accompany them to healthcare providers for any types of "women's problems." I was also frequently recruited to visit women who were sick in their homes or in the hospital. I was sought out to evacuate pregnant women with medical emergencies, like Rosario, to the hospital. Watching women attempt to navigate public, non-governmental organizations (NGOs) and private health-care systems and being present when families interpreted illness and negotiated healthcare choices was at many times painful for me to witness, but invaluable as a learning tool.

My life and experiences in Santa Cruz form the basis of this ethnography, yet this is really a far more comprehensive look at efforts to decrease maternal mortality in Sololá. Obtaining a detailed understanding of how this campaign affected people on an everyday level meant that I had to incorporate many sites and many methods into this study.

From the day I arrived I tried to integrate myself as much as possible into the Safe Motherhood campaign. I traveled frequently around the health district to which Santa Cruz belonged. I learned about State-provided prenatal care by observing women who came to health posts for prenatal visits, traveling with Ministry of Health–contracted health workers to neighboring villages that lacked a health post to help with prenatal efforts, and going on house calls to deliver prenatal care to pregnant women who had not come into the clinic on their own. I also participated in the meetings between *iyoma*, as the local midwives were called, and the Ministry of Health throughout the district.[19]

There was always a lot to be done in Sololá to improve Safe Motherhood, and on the departamental level, I stayed abreast of what the Ministry of Health and the NGOs were trying to do. This involved going to a lot of meetings where, in addition to the business of the

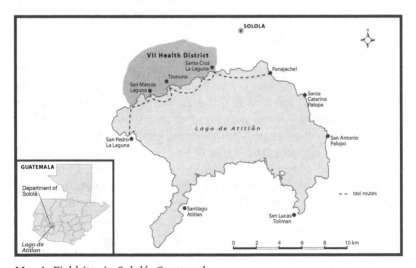

MAP 1. Fieldsites in Sololá, Guatemala

day, we always had the opportunity to eat lunch and drink coffee. I very much appreciated and enjoyed forming professional relationships with colleagues, the vast majority of whom had much more expertise in the area of maternal health than I did. I was able to call on these relationships for the help that I needed—from explanations about medical particulars of certain maternal deaths to advice about designing interview protocols.

During my second year of fieldwork attempts to improve the quality of emergency obstetric care at the hospital became much more important to my work. I participated in the doctor training sessions where the latest protocol for obstetric emergencies was introduced and where we practiced manual actions on the torsos of mannequins. I made daily trips to the hospital for two and a half months to see what happened when a woman came to the hospital with an obstetric emergency. I spent many days sitting in the general emergency room (ER) and then the obstetric (OB) section watching interactions between doctors, nurses, patients, and their families. I also followed patients from the ER to the maternity ward and to the operating room. Informally, I interacted with hospital workers at all levels, from the janitorial staff to the social workers and record keepers. Nevertheless, I call my activities in the hospital "observation" because I did not actually participate in providing medical care, nor did I advocate for the patients.

When I originally designed this study I assumed that the primary interactions that I would observe in the obstetric ER would be between the healthcare providers and the women themselves.[20] After observing the ER for one week I realized that this assumption was completely unfounded. There was very little conversation between patients and the medical staff. In fact, constructing the patient as singular denied the social reality of the hospital. The few unaccompanied individuals I saw in any part of the ER were picked up off the street by the firemen and all of these cases attested to some sort of social pathology—men who were drunk and passed out blocking the road and a woman beaten by her husband and then thrown out of the house and into the street. There was no case of anyone in the OB section of the ER ever coming in alone, whether they had a scheduled appointment or were unscheduled. I, therefore, quickly had to amend my research ethics permissions to include family members in the study.

While I ran around Sololá I tried to formally interview as many people as possible. One of my primary focuses concerned what happened in a homebirth when a woman had an obstetric emergency and, closely related to that, why a woman remained at home instead of seeking biomedical care. To discover women who had remained at home during an emergency, I carried out two courses of "village" interviews in Santa Cruz and two surrounding Kaqchikel Villages. These village interviews consisted of a demographic survey that included a reproductive history, information on the use of different health resources, and educational and household information. I then had a number of open-ended questions that dealt directly with women's feelings about using the hospital for emergency obstetric care, assessments of risk, understandings of biomedical treatments, etc. All of these interviews were completed with the assistance of a trained field assistant. Because most women had no experience with interviews and disliked dry questioning, we tried to make the interviews as conversation-like as possible. The field assistant would ask the questions, which she had largely memorized, and I would take notes on the woman's answer, interjecting if I wanted more information about a situation. The longest interviews took an hour and a half; the shortest, about twenty minutes. All of these interviews were of course completed in Kaqchikel. Most participants were revisited after six months for a follow-up interview. Also, if it seemed after writing up an interview that a relevant detail had been left out, women were revisited. I completed 122 random interviews with women and 13 non-random interviews with men. Unlike the random sample of women, I chose the male participants sheerly because they were loitering in a public space (like outside of the barber's shop, at the dock, or in the center of town). While it would have been nice to add men to my random interview sample in the village, this was impractical as most men work all day Monday through Saturday afternoon. Sunday is their only day off, and those who are not in church are playing basketball or soccer. There was no time except for the evening to find men in their homes (a condition necessary for my random survey), and I could not ask a field assistant to work nights, nor was I comfortable walking around and knocking on strangers' doors at those hours. Thus, the village interviews with men that I did get, I got on weekends. All of the male participants come from Santa Cruz.

To better understand why women did end up in the hospital, I made thirty-three audio recordings of healthcare worker–client interactions in the ER and had a follow-up interview with all but one of the woman recorded.[21] While I was able to communicate with most of them by speaking Kaqchikel or Spanish, either neighboring patients or a midwife helped me conduct the interviews with monolingual speakers of K'iche' and Tz'utujil. While I administered the same demographic survey that I used in the village, the follow-up questions concerned the decision-making process to send the patient to the hospital and her experience once she arrived. In addition to interviewing the recorded patients, I interviewed ten husbands, four midwives, three family groups, two mothers, one father-in-law, and one brother who accompanied the patients. Again, I concentrated on understanding the decision-making process that led up to their presence in the hospital, as well as their perception and understanding of what had occurred since they arrived. As families always bring at least one Spanish speaker with them to the hospital, communication was never an issue in these interviews. In many instances I ran into and chatted with family members over several days.

The multiple sites and diverse research methodologies have been crucial to this work. I have been able to present a far more holistic understanding of why maternal mortality was not decreasing in Sololá than I would have had I restricted myself to a "village study" or decided to just concentrate on the Safe Motherhood campaign itself. This work also intends to take the discussion of why women are reluctant to use the state-provided healthcare to another level by presenting data that could not be gathered through interviews or surveys. My use of audio recordings has allowed me to enrich our understanding of how structural issues, such as race, ethnicity, and multilingualism, are enacted in the delivery of healthcare, making it profoundly uncomfortable for disenfranchised Maya. I use this rich data to construct a detailed picture of how women, families, and *iyoma* are motivated to seek out certain types of care and why health workers are motivated to shape the care they offer in particular ways. As I describe in the following chapters, the Safe Motherhood campaign in Sololá rests on top of this maneuvering, sometimes intersecting with the needs and desires of the involved parties, yet at other times remaining completely disconnected.

Outline of Chapters

This book is divided into six different chapters. Chapters 1 and 2 examine the two settings for birth: the home and the hospital. I begin chapter 1 by exploring village life in the Guatemalan highlands where I lived. With that context in hand, I focus on the everyday practices surrounding pregnancy and childbirth in Santa Cruz. I analyze these practices to show how childbirth is an important local site

where kin ties are formed, which creates and reinstantiates mutually constituted, relational subjectivities. This chapter highlights the
costs of policies that seek to move birth out of the home and into
the hospital. Chapter 2 takes us directly to the obstetric emergency
room, where we follow the admission of one woman whose family
brings her to the hospital with an obstetric complication. A micro-
level analysis of the interaction between the family and the nurse in
the obstetric ER helps reveal the everyday terms upon which Safe
Motherhood's message of "skilled care" is propagated. The micro-
analysis provides a link between the global Safe Motherhood campaign and how health workers use policy to reorganize daily practices related to childbirth in order to promote particular "modern"
subjectivities that can remake Guatemala. Ultimately the chapter
poignantly illustrates why seeking care can be profoundly uncomfortable for poor, indigenous Maya.

Chapters 3 and 4 take a closer looks at the impact of policy in helping to prevent maternal mortality. Chapter 3 puts the Guatemalan
Safe Motherhood efforts in conversation with the global initiative,
by outlining how the Safe Motherhood campaign in Guatemala has
followed the contours of larger, global Safe Motherhood. It enriches
our understanding of how the design of the local Sololá campaign
is linked to a global initiative, and how both assume a western, autonomous subject as the client of the campaign. In this chapter I use
the notion of spin to illustrate how the terms upon which the global
campaign has been waged have actually impeded our ability to decrease maternal mortality. Chapter 4 focuses on the rejection of particular Mayan subjects by the Guatemalan healthcare system. I trace
how this rejection occurs at all levels: in health worker–client interactions, in hospital policy, and in mandated policy from the Ministry
of Health. This chapter helps highlight the local narratives available
in post–civil war Guatemala into which the discourses of the global
Safe Motherhood campaign ultimately were incorporated.

Chapter 5 explores the everyday lives of the Kaqchikel men and
women who live in places that suffer such high rates of maternal
mortality. The theme of violence frames this chapter and I argue that
violence is paramount both to understanding the history and on-
going daily experiences in Guatemala. I use violence as an entrée
into my field site, showing how social organization and economic
resources available to villagers have been shaped, at least in part,
by the violence. In my view this legacy of violence is critical to the
prejudice and rejection certain Mayan subjects/citizens experience
in Guatemala. Many particularly middle and upper class Guatema-

lans see the ethnic divisions of the past as a motivator for continued violence. They conceptualize the way forward as a "modern," democratic, uniform Guatemala where the populace shares important values (education, health, hard work, small families, etc.). I tie the positive reception of global Safe Motherhood within the national health systems to the fact that it both represents and embodies this new, "modern" Guatemala.

Chapter 6 looks at how the Safe Motherhood campaign gets translated at the village level, and what this means to the practices outlined in chapter 1. This discussion brings to the fore different ways of viewing problems in pregnancy and childbirth. The local Safe Motherhood campaign betrays the bias of the global campaign and views maternal mortality as a biomedical problem, while in Santa Cruz, physical problems during pregnancy and birth are generally considered manifestations of underlying social problems, such as a poor relationship with God resulting from sin. These differing etiologies lead to different means of addressing problems: while health workers want women to receive biomedical attention, villagers place a premium on dealing with and resolving social ills.

As my Kaqchikel informants pointed out time and time again, for the woman who is pregnant, birth is what Victor Turner (1957) would call a *liminal* state. "Täq xatel libre," they say—literally meaning "maybe you will leave free," and figuratively meaning "maybe you will get out alive, but maybe not." Birth is also one of the few areas where ethnographers have achieved a deep intimacy with their subjects. That same intimacy is present in the ethnographer's experience of studying death during birthing. This ethnography firmly places us in the difficult, intimate spaces where mothers who should have lived die.

Chapter 1

LIFE, BIRTH, AND DEATH
IN THE VILLAGE

Life in Santa Cruz

When I first arrived in Santa Cruz I wondered how living in the shadows of three enormous volcanoes for generations would impact people in the village. The longer I stayed in Santa Cruz, the more I began to regard the volcanoes as pictures on the wall—what was far more relevant in organizing our lives was that we lived perched high on a mountainside. The terrain leading to Santa Cruz was so steep that no road had been built connecting the village to the outside world. Rather, to get to Santa Cruz, you had to come by boat, and then walk about five hundred meters uphill. One pick-up truck had been ferried over to the village some years before and it was the only available mechanized, albeit expensive, transport between the dock and the village itself. A thriving local economy of porters had developed since carrying weight up the hill was a challenge even for the young and able-bodied. The steep landscape also corralled people in the village—people wouldn't walk the hill unless necessary, or would refuse to walk it midday. For those un-accustomed to the terrain it was particularly grueling. Santa Cruz is the municipal seat, so visitors from other villages were obligated to trek up from the shore to conduct their official business (registering births, deaths, obtaining identity cards, paying taxes, etc.).

A lot of my time in Santa Cruz was spent in the central square. On the north end of the square was the centuries old Catholic church. To the south stood the new municipal building and a public

clothes-washing site. To the west was the health post established by
the Ministry of Health. The east side of the square was predomi-
nated by educational buildings: the preschool, library, and elementary school. The voter registration office was housed next to the
library. The square itself had been renovated and was now a multi-
use court, and was, consequently, one of most popular social hang-
outs in town. During recess hours, after school, after the workday,
and on weekends the court filled with basketball and soccer games.
If you weren't at the square to socialize then you often had to walk
through it to get where you were going. The only other public buildings in town were the *Juez de Paz* [Judge of the Peace] and churches.
Santa Cruz hosted three Evangelical churches, and a fourth was being built as I left.

Because Santa Cruz is built on a small plateau, the ability of the
town to expand outward is limited by the steep hillsides. After becoming more familiar with the neighboring villages, I was surprised
by how much Cruceños had embraced densification to make the
most of their limited space. The Kaqchikel word *jay* translates into
both "room" and "house," mirroring the fact that traditional family
compounds consist of several independent, one-room houses positioned around a courtyard, usually with a separate house for cooking. Yet one strategy that people in Santa Cruz adopted was to build
one-room houses that shared a wall. Sometimes newer structures
even connected rooms from the inside of the house. Another strategy for the more well-off was to build from concrete block and rebar. Inevitably, one could see metal rods sticking out of the roof that
allowed the future expansion of the house upward. Unlike the other
villages around the lake, very few houses still existed that were constructed out of cane poles bound together, with mud packed in between the crevices to form a wall. The majority of villagers use the
locally manufactured adobe brick and wooden shutters. Some of
these houses had tile floors while others had polished concrete and
glass windows. The older styles of tile or straw roofs had disappeared
in favor of corrugated metal. The metal was cheaper, easier to transport, and not as likely to cave in during an earthquake. It did, however, fly away in heavy winds, which could easily be a problem.
Nevertheless, stories about running around in the dark and trying
to find one's roof did garner laughs the next day.

In Santa Cruz, densification was needed not necessarily because
of expanding nuclear families, but because children married and ideally brought their spouses back to live with their parents. According
to the door-to-door census performed in 2000 by the auxiliary nurse

working in the Santa Cruz health post, 240 heads of family were registered in the village with an average of 4.8 persons per house. A full 24 percent of all houses were female-headed, and these families had an average of 3.5 persons compared to 5.2 persons for a male-headed household. In addition, 50 percent of the population was under the age of 18. Since people tended to marry within the village, almost everyone was related to everyone else.

As the population increased while space remained constant, the question of what to do with waste became more and more problematic. The fields that people used to squat in to defecate or urinate were eliminated. Those who could afford it tried to put some sort of bathroom into their compound. According to the census 71 percent of houses (60 percent for female-headed) were recorded as having "adequate" facilities for the disposal of excrement, which in most cases meant a pit toilet, and in a few cases might have meant a septic tank. The other 29 percent, I found out over the course of two years, availed themselves in the houses of relatives, sought out now urban patches of land that weren't built on, or in the worst case, used public paths when no one was looking. One man frequently complained to me about the stink that wafted into his house from the undeveloped piece of land abutting his compound. He felt that he was living in a toilet. He was considering developing the land or putting up barbwire to stop his neighbors from defecating there.

But human waste was not the only problem that the tight space created for Cruceños. There was no "trash boat" that would carry away waste. Instead, the strategy seemed to be throwing trash over cliffs or throwing it into a steep stream bed, where the first rains would wash it away into the lake. Officially, only one cliff was the sanctioned dump. When you had trash you could tie it up in a plastic bag and give a passing child a few cents to dispose of it for you. In general, though, most of us burned our trash several times a week. Yet as more and more people occupied the spaces of the village, once the rains started, unofficial dumps started to flow into family compounds. The trash "problem," people told me, was relatively new, because only in the last fifteen years had plastic come onto the scene. Before that all purchases were either wrapped in organic matter, like meat in banana leaves, or in newspaper, which could easily be burned or eventually breaks down. The fact that throwing things onto the ground was a common, not contraband, behavior might also have aggravated the trash problem. For example, much waste produced during a meal, like banana leaves or husks used to wrap corn dough, are thrown directly onto the floor and then swept up after eating. Throwing trash on the ground and walking away was not frowned upon unless the trash blew into someone's compound.

Despite the fact that the situation was more complicated, most older Cruceños viewed Santa Cruz as a village of agriculturalists. Indeed, one day I met a frustrated surveyor in the town square who reported that at house after house he asked people what they did and they responded that they were agriculturalists. Then he would ask them how much land they had and they would say none. He would then have to ask several more questions until their method of income generation finally fit into one of the boxes he could mark. Every family in Santa Cruz used to have access to land, but in the middle of the last century collectively owned land was carved up and privatized. As the interests of outsiders in the lake grew, villagers sold off the flat lands by the shore that they used for their crops.[1] Now many families are left without any land to farm at all. Regardless of how many families own land, every family knows that corn is of central importance to their survival. The village is surrounded by *milpa* [fields of corn]. To plant the milpa, a field must be "cleaned" using a machete to chop down all of the growth, after which it is left fallow to allow the weeds to die, and then the corn seeds are planted in small mounds. As the corn begins to grow it must be cleaned again of new weeds. Eventually the milpa can be harvested. In Santa Cruz, people frequently plant squashes and beans in their milpa, though they generally refer to it as only corn. On the steep, unterraced mountainsides, yields are poor and corn is never exported from Santa Cruz for sale.

The steepness and cramped space of Santa Cruz did not mean, however, that Cruceños had no food stuffs to cultivate to abundance. Fruit trees, like avocados, fit well into the landscape. The trees around the village were individually owned but there was a local market in leasing a tree for a season. The municipality of Santa Cruz was renowned for the quality of its *jocote,* another tree fruit, and thus they commanded a high price at markets in Panajachel or Sololá. Bananas presented a similar case. Many people had bananas planted both in their courtyards and on any other land they might have had. Bananas could always be taken to the market and sold for some extra cash in one day. Many of the bananas grown in Santa Cruz were heirloom or non-commercial varieties [*casera*], and thus they commanded a higher price than the left-over Chiquita bananas that got bussed up from the coast. Perhaps the most notable export from Santa Cruz was the coffee. Since coffee grows well on steep slopes, much of the land too steep to cultivate otherwise had been planted in coffee. Unlike many other villages around the lake, there was no mechanized way to process coffee in the village. In the past families would spend several weeks around the harvests doing the job by hand. In recent years, however, the harvests were sold after picking, but before processing, to outsiders. Finally, many men and children in Santa Cruz spent a significant amount of time fishing. Rights to fish in the lake with a net from a canoe were passed down in families between male kin. You could see men in canoes out every morning either catching small fish or diving for small crabs, which they could sell locally. Little boys would fish with a piece of line directly from docks, bringing anything they caught home to their families. Since the sweetness of the fish and crabs in Santa Cruz was well known, middlemen (or in this case middle women) came to Santa Cruz once a week to buy fish and take it back to their own villages to sell. Regardless of the fact that each compound might no longer cultivate a piece of land with corn, agricultural activity was commonly part of people's everyday lives.

The income that people generated from agricultural activities was, however, usually a supplement to their "day job." Some of the more lucrative jobs in Santa Cruz for men were foreman/contractor, tailor, shop owner, real estate dealer, pastor, and owner or driver of a boat taxi. Some of the less lucrative but more plentiful jobs were day laborer agriculturalists, assistant (*ayudante*) (to a "*guardian*," or skilled

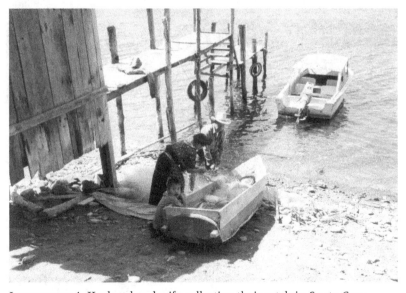

ILLUSTRATION 4. Husband and wife collecting their catch in Santa Cruz

construction worker), harvester and seller of firewood, and porter. The village also had one car driver and one barber.

A variety of other jobs were available to women who wanted to earn extra cash by working outside of the home. One of the most difficult jobs that was predominantly performed by women was harvester and seller of firewood. As deforestation became more and more of a problem in the municipality of Santa Cruz, women had to walk farther and farther away to find wood. Conversely, this meant that they had to carry full bundles of wood on their backs from farther distances. Another traditional job for a woman was to work as a *"muchacha."*[2] During births, deaths, and other special occasions, families would frequently need the assistance of someone who could prepare food, serve guests, keep things clean, and just generally help out. Muchachas were also sought out by *tiendas* [small stores], as they had to be paid far less than a man for doing equal work.

Women in Santa Cruz were extremely talented and well-renowned weavers. Women from other towns would visit to place special orders for a *huipil,* the traditional blouse that women wore. Cruceñas also made money doing *bordado* [hand-stitching]. They decorated cloth both for other locals, and again, for outsiders who came seeking their services. While neither of these activities was particularly lucrative, they were convenient as a woman could work at home during any extra time she might have.

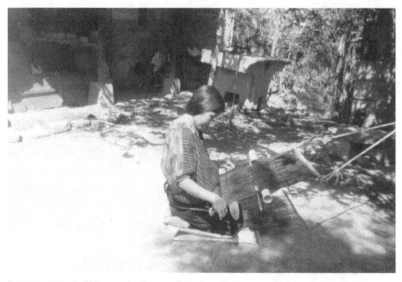

ILLUSTRATION 5. Weaver in Santa Cruz.

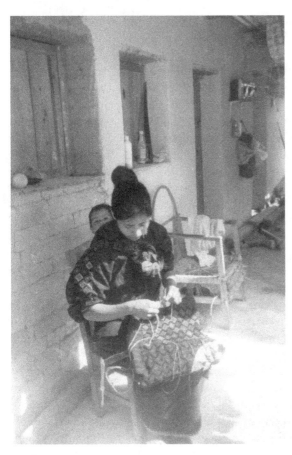

ILLUSTRATION 6.
Woman hand stitch-
ing a huiple.

The influx of gringos[3] along the shore heavily impacted women's ability to earn cash. Many weavers attempted to sell their wears directly to tourists and a few had branched out from traditional cloths to hand-woven purses and scarves. While these products commanded a better price, during the rainy season, when tourism was slower, it was difficult to survive on this alone. New jobs for women had also been created; the four hotels for tourists that were on the shore were predominantly staffed by females, who cooked the meals and cleaned the rooms. Women working these jobs made as much in four hours as a man doing agricultural day labor for another villager made in eight. Women also sought out opportunities to wash clothes or clean the houses of the local gringo chalet owners. The cleaning jobs were frequently done by married women with families both because a husband who worked at the house usually got his wife the job and because women could bring their children with them. The hotel jobs, on the other hand, were most normally sought out by younger, unmarried women. Several of the hotel workers had left their jobs after getting married since their husbands said that they couldn't fulfill their home duties and work the hours the hotels demanded at the same time. The wage labor for women, however, opened up possibilities for female-headed households to be economically viable.

Finally, a number of children worked in Santa Cruz, though there were only a few jobs they regularly performed, and all were badly paid. One of the main sources of income for kids was carrying goods up the hill. Renting the car for a trip from the dock to the village cost a flat rate of 25 Q,[4] but if one had only a few things it was far cheaper to hire a porter than to rent the car. Cases of soda and beer or propane gas tanks are good examples of smaller things that needed to go up to the village. Children's work was not as highly valued as that of men, and when a load could be carried by either, a child would earn less for equal work. Many families hiring a porter, therefore, preferred to hire a child over an adult. With the influx of gringos, children now crowded the dock hoping to be able to carry a tourist's backpack from the boat to a hotel. Two other infrequent sources of cash for kids were disposing of trash or running errands. Gringos frequently used children as a local mail service, paying them a postage fee to hand deliver a message. It is important to note that while many men and women did work for cash, only the poorest of the poor children had to work. Many of these were illiterate, and their parents needed their incomes to supplement the family. They, therefore, were not able to go to school.

Yet even those who could go to school were frequently challenged to get a good education. Most of the village schools on the west side of Lake Atitlán (like Santa Cruz) were staffed by teachers from the town of San Pedro La Laguna. San Pedro boasted a secondary school that certified teachers, and since there was such easy access to the profession, a disproportionate number of Pedranos chose to be teachers.[5] The positions at local schools in San Pedro quickly filled, so Pedranos applied to work in different schools around the lake. With a water taxi service available between San Pedro and the villages on the west side of the lake (like Santa Cruz), teachers could still live at home with their families and commute to work. What this meant for the schools on the west side of the lake was that their teachers were in general waiting to take the next boat out. Schools in the area were hopelessly under funded and since few villagers were formally educated, the schools needed teachers who were leaders and interested in building the community. But parents complained that many Pedranos had no interest in improving the schools in which they taught—rather teachers tried to spend the absolute minimum amount of time possible at work. Most Pedranos were seen as commuters whose community was elsewhere. This inspired little confidence in local schools.

Despite this bleak picture the elementary school in Santa Cruz, called Tecun Uman, boasted several unique advantages over, for example, the school in Tzununá (the only other village in the municipality that had the same population of youth). The Santa Cruz school profited from having very good directors over the past years. One of the first Cruceños to graduate with his teaching credential was hired on to teach at the local elementary. After several years he rose to the position of director. The implicit knowledge of the community that he possessed by being Cruceño significantly contributed to the success of the school. He made it a personal campaign to get all children enrolled in school and he visited houses where children were not attending to converse with the parents about the necessity of literacy and education in present-day Guatemala. As an insider he knew who had children and where they lived. He also was able to visit people's houses without them feeling like this was an "official" visit—a feat not easily accomplished by an outsider. In 2002, a new director who was a Pedrano was appointed. This director also was extremely devoted to the education of the pupils, willing to work long hours and he even slept in Santa Cruz if need be. As luck would have it, both directors got along well and were like minded in terms of values and pedagogy.

Elementary education in Santa Cruz has also been significantly impacted by the presence of foreigners. Many of the gringos in the chalet community on the shore either are or were teachers in their home countries, so working with the elementary school seemed like an obvious way for them to contribute to the community. In 1998 the gringos founded an organization called Amigos de Santa Cruz to offer support to the schools and students. It was incorporated as a 501(c)3 under US law in 2001. Working with the director of the school and the Ministry of Education in Sololá, Amigos was able to coordinate the resources going into the school and offer significant financial support. Tecun Uman was one of the few public schools that provided full scholarships for every pupil—this meant that every child received textbooks, notebooks, pencils, paper, etc. To improve the pedagogy, Amigos made an agreement with the Ministry of Education to supplement the school budget and increase the number of teachers hired per year, decreasing the number of children per classroom, and Tecun Uman students had access to a computer lab and the school boasted a secretary and a copy machine. Students also received a nutritious lunch or a snack. Though resources do not necessarily translate into education, many parents were more willing to send their children to a school where they received "gifts," then one that was completely under funded.

As the description of all of the work and obligations portends, life in Santa Cruz was incredibly busy. We were woken up every morning at dawn by one of the Evangelical congregants greeting the new day and praying over a portable loud speaker. Cruceños who had to go to town would be gathered around the dock waiting to go with the first boat at 6:30 AM. Those tending the fields or collecting firewood would have been long gone, hoping to get home before the midday sun. Those still at home would be making tortillas and coffee, and getting ready for the day. At 7:30 most paid jobs and school began. Women who remained in the village during the day always had numerous chores to attend to: the compound needed to be swept; laundry needed to be done; corn would need to be prepared and soaked in lye for tomorrow's tortillas; pre-soaked corn would need to be drained, loaded into a plastic tub, and taken to the mill, where, if one waited too long there was inevitably a line; once the corn was ground, tortillas or *tamalitos* would need to be prepared, and any other cooking would need to be done. When possible, women would leave enough time to socialize with their kin or to attend a church activity. From midday onward, villagers would return from the fields or the woods or their trip to the city. Around 3:30 phalanxes of men could be seen climbing the paths back to the village. The square would then fill up with people playing sports and socializing. This was doubly so on the weekends. Despite all of the hustle and bustle, in Santa Cruz it was unusual to leave a compound completely unattended. Latches were more to secure a door than to lock it and windows always provided an alternate entrance. The population of Santa Cruz was small and families were large, so very few weeks passed when there was not a death, baptism, confirmation, marriage, or some other event that one was invited to attend. This meant that in addition to all of the normal daily work, people were frequently planning and preparing for some sort of ritual occasion.

Yet socializing often brought to the fore one of the scourges of Santa Cruz: alcohol. Very few women in Santa Cruz drank, but drinking was the curse of many men. Walking along the paths during the day it was not uncommon to step over men lying on the ground, passed out and filthy. Unlike Catholics, who condone drinking in principle, Evangelicals derided any contact with alcohol. Yet many Cruceños, Evangelical or not, were actively opposed to drinking because it could be persuasively argued that drinking, as practiced in Santa Cruz, was deleterious. Drinking was social, in that it happened mostly in public spaces and there were many marked occasions, such as payday and celebrations, where the point was for men to gather to drink. However, "social drinking"—i.e., having just one or two drinks then stopping—was not the norm; most men who drank continued until they were very drunk or passed out.[6] Many women, like Rosario, objected to their husbands' excessive drinking. It was both bad for his health and for his work life. Drinking could increase family violence. A drunken husband was not able to be responsible and drunken men were more likely to do stupid things like get in fights or have affairs. They were also more likely to be robbed. In a village where money was particularly tight, many women had to compete with their husbands' drinking habits to be able to pay the bills and feed their children. In short, drinking heavily impacted all of the family.

Birth in the Village

As I mentioned previously, my training in Kaqchikel was through immersion in Santa Cruz. Because I knew that I needed vocabulary related to birth, I asked my language teacher to tell me generally what an ideal childbirth was like. I followed my method of recording and transcribing what he said. While I mastered the vocabulary and grammar, understanding what was "ideal" about this narrative was not so straightforward. Debates that had surrounded !Kung birth threw into relief how non-descriptive "ideal" could be. Nancy Howell (1979) reported that the ideal !Kung birth was one where a woman birthed alone. But the existence of this ideal certainly did not translate into many !Kung women achieving it.[7] When I finally did start interviewing women and asking them about their births, I realized that the "ideal" birth narrative my teacher told me about roughly described many of the births I heard about, yet, there were inevitable divergences. Why did some of the women I talked to recapitulate his version (though with far more details), others only recapitulate it some of the time, and still others have birth experiences that were more similar to my experience having children in a hospital in the United States than to anyone I had talked to in the village?

That story, which constituted my introduction to birth in Kaq-chikel villages that I worked in, frames the next part of this chapter. The ideal birth story most closely fit the experiences of young, married first-time mothers, and most greatly diverged from older women who were the heads of their own compounds. Why would the ideal birth be the one representing that of a young daughter-in-law rather than a senior woman? From a western feminist perspective that emphasizes choice in birth,[8] certainly quite the opposite was true. In fact, senior women frequently appeared to have more individual choice and control over younger women's birth than the young women did themselves.

How do we make sense of the emphasis on young, married, first-time mothers' births as representing some sort of ideal? I argue that young, married women's births are represented as ideal because they represent the best exemplar of how birth binds people together. Rather than the ideal birth being represented by the comfort of the woman during parturition, the ideal narrative highlights the birth event as a primary location for the performance and instantiation of kinship ties—not as one might assume between a mother and her child, but rather ties that bind a woman to her affinal family.[9] Santa Cruz generally follows a pattern of patrilocal residence, where a young married couple moves into a groom's family's compound. As described below in the birth narrative, pregnancy and birth provide rich and meaningful opportunities for mothers-in-law to act like mothers-in-law to their daughters-in-law and vice versa, and husbands to behave as husbands to wives, etc. The result of these performances is that a woman is woven into the fabric of her new family. In a small town where almost everyone is related to everyone else, family forms the main social group. In his story about the ideal, my teacher made obvious the primary importance of birth as a site for forging and strengthening kin relations.

I next present the ideal birth narrative to highlight all of the opportunities that pregnancy and birth offer to tie people together. I then look at the experiences of those whose births were not at all ideal according to this standard and analyze these stories in relation to kin building.

My Language Teacher's Narrative of an "Ideal" Pregnancy and Birth

When a woman discovers she is pregnant she tells her husband. Her husband, in consultation with his own mother, then chooses a midwife who he calls on at her house, inviting her to visit his pregnant wife. They agree on a day during the following week that the midwife will come, and on this evening the family lights the *t'uj*.[10] The pregnant woman enters the *t'uj*, where the midwife comes and finds her. The midwife examines the woman to make sure that she and the fetus are healthy. Each time that the midwife attends to the pregnant woman, the woman's family serves her coffee and bread and gives her tortillas to take home as a token of their gratitude. These visits continue, perhaps monthly at first, and then weekly as the pregnancy progresses.

The midwife is in charge of relieving the discomforts of pregnancy, which she accomplishes through her skills at massage and a variety of teas for nausea, exhaustion, swelling, or headaches. Later in the pregnancy one of the primary responsibilities of the midwife is to monitor the position of the baby and manipulate that position so that the baby engages head first. If a fetus is not positioned correctly she will gently massage the abdomen to turn it. This may only take one session; it may mean that the midwife must return several times a day for a few days until it is turned; or she may have to manipulate it every day for a few weeks. Late in the pregnancy the midwife will give the family a list of things that they need to buy for the birth such as oil for massaging the abdomen, soap for the midwife to wash her hands, and herbs for teas. The midwife will ask the family to always have boiled water and a towel available.

When a woman goes into labor she sends a messenger to get the midwife and to alert her husband if he is absent. A woman usually gives birth in the room where she and her husband sleep. In addition to the woman, her husband, and the midwife, the birth will be attended by at least her mother or mother-in-law and perhaps both sets of parents and parents-in-law, her sisters, her grandmother, or aunt, and perhaps an older daughter. During labor the woman does not disrobe, but loosens her huipil. The midwife ties a belt around the pregnant woman's upper abdomen, the purpose of which is to constrict the area enough to not allow the baby to return to the womb. As the birth progresses and the baby moves down and engages the pelvic bone and, eventually, the birth canal, the belt is lowered. A woman in labor is free to stand up, walk around, squat, or lay down. When it is her time, the midwife will tell her to push. Traditionally, the husband squats behind the wife and holds her up while she births the baby. Many families hang ropes with handles from the rafters of their house that the couple can use for extra support. If the family has a bed, the woman positions herself on the bed.

If not, she and her husband position themselves on the floor over bedding and blankets. If a woman is having problems the midwife may massage her belly to help relieve the pain.

After the baby is born the mother is taken to the *t'uj*, where she will recover and be washed off with a bucket of hot water. The mother should then enjoy thirty days of repose (the first eight of which are spent in bed) with the infant before resuming her normal duties. Her husband hires a young woman to come to the house and do the cooking and cleaning. Friends and relatives will send chicken stews and tortillas. The midwife visits the woman every day and checks her and the baby. Eight days after the baby is born the parents will celebrate. The husband will go out and buy several large chickens in the market in Sololá to make stew and tortillas. He will hire women or his female relatives will help prepare the foods. They must make enough food to repay each of the friends and relatives who sent him food, ideally returning more than was received. Younger children are enlisted to carry bowls of stew and cloth bundles of tortillas to these families. He also must make food to pay the midwife. She is normally offered an entire three to five gallon kettle of stew that includes at least one large chicken and many tortillas.[11] She will come mid afternoon, clean the woman's room, enjoy a meal, and then take the rest of the food with her. On this day the family will also invite over special friends or relatives to celebrate the baby.

Performing Kinship, Defining Kinship

The value of my teacher's narrative of an ideal birth is not its typicality, but rather how it helps us understand how kin relations are forged and strengthened in this Kaqchikel community. The practices that surround pregnancy and birth demonstrate that the kin ties of in-laws are not taken for granted, but rather develop through everyday actions that forge relatedness. Daniela Peluso's work with Ese Eje, a group of indigenous Amazonians, helps us see how the ideal birth narrative describes these processes of kin-making: "Ese Eje continually shape and reaffirm relatedness … through the quality and reciprocity of acts of nurturance, care taking, cooperation and generosity" (Peluso 2003 as cited in Lepri 2005). Contracting the midwife demonstrates one such example of how relatedness is strengthened. On a practical level, by the time a woman gets pregnant she has known the midwives in the village all of her life, has undoubtedly been privy to her own relatives' discussions about the skill of each midwife, and has probably developed a closer relationship with the midwife her own family uses than with the others. Nevertheless, it is her husband in consultation with his mother who chooses and alerts a midwife. The immediate responsiveness and plan-making concerning a daughter-in-law's comfort and safety demonstrate how her new family cares for her. Their financial support in paying for a midwife demonstrates their generosity toward their daughter-in-law and giving her an eight-day recovery period shows how her family wants to nurture her back to health. These examples also demonstrate the importance of respect, hierarchy, and responsibility in defining kin ties. Deferring to one's husband and allowing him to make the choice of appropriate midwife is part of being a respectful wife. Deferring to one's parents' choice of a midwife is part of a respectful attitude toward them. Parents or parents-in-law ultimately are responsible for making good choices for their children and children-in-law.

The fact that the ideal birth required the cooperation of daughters-in-law to be successful was highlighted during interviews in the stories that women told me about midwives that their in-laws had chosen. One younger woman, Josefa, expressed her disdain for the midwife her mother-in-law picked, who attended the births of her first two children. Josefa said that during both of her births, the midwife insisted that she start pushing before she was ready. At the first birth Josefa referred to herself as young and inexperienced, so she listened when the midwife told her to start to push. By the time she really had the urge to push Josefa was already exhausted. After the birth, she said that she suffered from an extremely sore stomach that she blamed on all of the pushing. When the midwife came to deliver Josefa's second child she told Josefa to push as soon as she got there. This time, however, Josefa told the midwife that she was not ready to push and that the midwife would have to wait until it was her time to really push. She told the midwife that they were paying her to be present, so she should have patience. There was no need to hurry through the birth.

This sort of story underscores that choice of midwife was not irrelevant, and that frequently women were not birthing with the midwife whom they preferred. Rather, women prioritized kin building activities like cooperating with their in-laws choices over insisting on a midwife whom they might like better. As this story demonstrates, cooperation and respect did not necessitate complete passivity. Later in this chapter I will take a closer look at some of the constraints that differentiated acceptable participation of a young parturient and her husband from unacceptable participation.

Making Family

As I came to understand the importance of pregnancy and birth
to family-making, I reviewed the interviews I did with Kaqchikel
women about their birthing experiences with renewed interest. I
asked myself how the stories that I heard adhered to or deviated
from the ideal. From that examination, certain patterns emerged.
For example, as I expected, mothers-in-law, in particular, almost
uniformly make a point of being present when a new daughter-
in-law gave birth. Yet I was quite surprised when I found that 3
women of 121 whom I interviewed reported that they had birthed
completely alone—no husband to hold them up, no in-law to run
and get help, no mother to hold their hand. But looking at the specifics of each of these less-than-ideal births helps us further understand the significance of pregnancy and birth to strengthening kin
relations.

Two of the women who reported having solitary births told me
very similar stories. In each case it was their last baby who was born
without anyone else around, and both told me that they had birthed
alone quite by mistake. In each situation, the woman reported that
she had been working in the house when her labor pains became
intense, but since everyone happened to be out doing other things
she had no one to call on to alert the midwife. In each case the
woman also said that the labor was strong and quick—so quick that
the birth was over before she had a chance to tell anyone what was
happening.

The third woman to birth alone was Mercedes. She told me that
she first got pregnant when she was 16, shortly after her mother
had died, and when she was the only child at home with her father.
After no male acknowledged paternity her dad moved her to an
isolated cabin out in the countryside, where he dedicated himself to
agriculture and she maintained the home. She had no contact with a
midwife. In fact, she had no contact with almost anyone while she
was pregnant. When it came time for her to give birth her father
was out in the fields. She was forced to go through labor and give
birth alone. The experience was quite frightening and she feared
that she would not survive. The baby, who was born without difficulties, did not live more than a year. After its death, Mercedes
moved back to her village and eventually got married. By the time
I interviewed her she was elderly and had birthed many more children, all of whom, she told me, were born under the watchful eyes
of a midwife.

How can we understand these stories of women who birthed alone, when the "ideal" is for pregnancy and birth to be used to cement the bonds between people? Essentially, these women birthed by themselves because in all three of the situations there was no new family to be made. The first two stories of the older women were told to me in passing, as mishaps that were laughable after the fact. These older women's reactions to their solitary births were consonant with their social positions—no other family member was to blame for these events, their birthing alone was not punishment, but rather a reflection of their seniority. There were no new bonds of kinship that needed to be formed during their parturitions. In comparison, decades later, Mercedes's story was still not laughable. Rather, her experience spoke to the difficult fact that single women for whom no male acknowledges paternity also do not have any "new" family into which to integrate.

In sum, women whose pregnancies lacked the opportunity to cement kin ties varied in diverse ways from the ideal birth. Age can solidify kinship ties, and as women achieve more seniority, their birthing events can become less scripted. Not surprisingly, fewer people attended the births of older women. Some of these women reported that they stopped alerting their husbands of their pregnancies. Some reported seeking out a midwife themselves. When young women got pregnant without having a partner claim responsibility, they experienced a lack of support. Conversely, a premium was placed on the first birth of a newly wed couple, since this event held the most opportunities to create social ties.

Social Context and Risk for Maternal Mortality

It became clear to me that the Safe Motherhood campaign was not unconnected to this idea that pregnancy and birth were significant family-making opportunities. The link was highlighted for me when I started to accompany Javiera on her rounds. Javiera, a doctor doing her six-month practicum with the government in a rural area of Sololá, was trying to increase prenatal screening by visiting pregnant women in their homes to perform exams. She spent many of her days walking around with the auxiliary nurse in one of the villages that I worked in, visiting women that the nurse knew were pregnant or suspected were pregnant. If a woman agreed to be examined, Javiera would pull out a new prenatal care chart and start a patient interview. Part of the World Health Organization's advocacy of Safe Motherhood has involved the international distribution of the prenatal care chart that Javiera used. The chart is supposed to help health workers assess if a woman is in a high-risk category for pregnancy or birthing complications by color-coding a woman's interview responses. Responses that fall into yellow boxes indicate a potential increase in risk. At the end of the interview the health worker can count the number of checked yellow boxes to assess potential risk. As Javiera and I walked from house to house we talked at length about why certain boxes were yellow.

The more time I spent talking to women in these villages about birth, the more I saw a divergence between patterns of risk associated with pregnancy and childbirth assumed in the WHO interview and patterns of risk that the local social context created. Three of the questions in particular seemed to illustrate how risk factors actually interacted to create distinctive risk patterns: How old are you? Is this your first child? And are you married? According to Javiera, while pregnancy-related complications such as retention of the placenta and hemorrhage equally strike women of all ages, other complications, such as birthing problems due to cephalopelvic disproportion and toxemia, strike younger women more frequently. Therefore, she asked about age. Care providers are interested in parity, or how many times a woman has given birth, because complications in previous pregnancies and deliveries help predict higher risk for the current pregnancies. A woman with no history of birthing will have no idea what to expect. Thus, Javiera asked if this was a woman's first child. Finally, married women are more likely to have access to the necessary financial resources required for a healthy pregnancy and birth, so she asked about marital status.

While these questions did identify factors that created a certain risk profile for women in Santa Cruz also, the logic of what sort of risk was created was different. Younger, married women with few children are in a particular position of risk, but not necessarily just for the reasons that the WHO assumes. Instead, ironically, the importance of pregnancy and birth for strengthening kin ties means that the more "ideal" one's birth is, the longer it is going to take to identify a birthing problem. In the "ideal" birth the extended family participates, lending physical, emotional, and spiritual support to the laboring woman. During this process kin ties are instantiated, particularly when a woman and her partner emphasize their respect for their parents. In this setting, having trouble, or even worse, openly identifying a problem, is a contentious activity that disrupts "ideal" birth. When a woman experiences trouble, she and/or her husband are frequently held responsible for the breakdown of the performance, both by themselves and by the rest of the family. In contrast to the hospital setting where no one blames a woman if she has a physiological problem, the failure to have an ideal homebirth is not blameless. An out-of-control physiology can be viewed as intentionally or unintentionally threatening social harmony. When the social stakes of having an ideal birth are high, participants from the woman herself, to the midwife, to family members should be reluctant to jump the gun on identifying any sort of obstetric complication. Depending on the problem, this delay in time may jeopardize the life of the woman.[12]

The claim that going to the hospital disrupts the cooperation that is integral to a successful "ideal" birth was illustrated by Tomasa's story. Tomasa, a woman in her late twenties and the mother of several healthy children, told me that she was very scared when she was pregnant with her first baby. She tried to talk to her mother about her own fear. She specifically asked if someone would get a doctor to operate on her if she was unable to get the baby out by herself. Her mother rejected the idea entirely. She told Tomasa that she would return to her mother-in-law's home and that one way or another, that baby would be born there, in her mother-in-law's house. She made clear that under no circumstances would Tomasa be going to the hospital.

My own sense of parenting is that when my children need reassurance I offer it, so I found Tomasa's mother's reaction somewhat cruel. Tomasa, however, did not see it that way. She seemed to view her early trepidations about childbirth the way I view my own trepidation to go down to the basement alone when I was little: as a silly childish fear. Of course her mother wasn't going to entertain Tomasa's fantasy, whether it was of bogeymen or non-existent obstetric complications. Tomasa told me that her mother only wanted the best for her, and the best would only come to Tomasa if she reciprocated her in-laws' nurturance and caring by birthing without complications at her in-laws' house.

Interestingly, this same association of a problem-free birth with familiar social harmony can also make it more likely for a family to seek biomedical care. Lisbeth married young and moved in with her husband's family. After she had four children her husband left her and went to live with another woman, yet Lisbeth and the children remained with her in-laws. She continued to have relations with her husband when he would come back and visit and she got pregnant by him two more times. In neither of these instances did her husband return to attend the births. However, her in-laws took responsibility for her pregnancies. They sought out the midwife, paid for the births and remained with her and supported her during each. Lisbeth's parents-in-law might not have been able to control their son's actions, but they certainly could control their own. Though Lisbeth's husband decided to abrogate his responsibilities to her, her in-laws made sure that she continued to be woven into the fabric of the family by taking care and nurturing Lisbeth through her pregnancies and births.

When Lisbeth got pregnant with twins and the first baby was stillborn and the second was stuck, both her midwife and in-laws were quick in deciding to move Lisbeth to the hospital. Since her husband had displayed decidedly bad faith in leaving his wife and his family, it was now incumbent on Lisbeth's in-laws to heal these wrongs by showing extra nurturance and generosity toward her. Thus, in Lisbeth's case, ignoring a birthing problem—rather than identifying one—would have been more threatening to kinship ties. Letting Lisbeth die in the throes of birth would have reflected very poorly on her in-laws. They could probably hear the accusations in their own minds as they watched a dead twin be born: first they ruined Lisbeth's life by producing a no-good son who didn't even fulfill his obligations to his wife, then they abrogated their own responsibility to take care of her by letting her die during birth. What kind of family were they? It's no surprise that her in-laws had already arranged for transport before they were certain whether or not Lisbeth would be able to push the second baby out.

As the WHO interview assumed, a lack of marriage could be associated with a dearth of resources necessary for a healthy pregnancy and birth. According to the 2000 door-to-door census performed by the auxiliary nurse, female-headed households did not enjoy the same level of health-related facilities. As discussed, fewer female-headed households enjoyed the presence of a bathroom. In addition, this census documented that 80 percent of houses overall in Santa Cruz had their own sources of running water in the house, while only 62 percent of female-headed households did. Those who did not have access to water in the house had to depend on community taps or wells and one female-headed household reported using only river water.

While this information confirms the comparative poverty of unmarried women, a more nuanced analysis is needed to understand how marital status can actually modulate both risk and protection. Like in many North American communities, a young woman who gets pregnant and bears her first child without marrying is frequently stigmatized. As the WHO would suspect, young, unmarried, pregnant woman have a very hard time receiving any economic or emotional resources during their pregnancy or for their birth. If a woman is pregnant and has no husband, who is going to pay the midwife for her visits? If the family is too embarrassed to call the midwife, who is going to give her money to travel to the doctor? Who is going to buy her the extra and nutritious foods that she needs to maintain her health during her pregnancy (and when she is breast feeding)? Who is going to pay for the baby clothes and the diapers? Parents are frequently upset when young, unmarried daughters become pregnant because they feel that it conflicts with their own child-rearing. As one father who had a pregnant, single daughter complained to me, he had his own children at home and his first responsibility was in raising them. His daughter couldn't even take care of herself. How was she going to provide for a new baby? He was angry at being put in this position and declared that his daughter was not a good person who could be trusted. In these conditions any pregnancy-related problems that a young woman might be experiencing often go unrecognized or ignored.

But illegitimate pregnancy puts young, unmarried women at additional risk for violence. During my fieldwork, a woman two villages over was apparently beaten unconscious by her father due to her illegitimate pregnancy. Alva was a single, professional, Evangelical woman who, at 25, was quickly approaching spinsterhood. When she became pregnant she immediately went and told her boyfriend what had happened. She was quite distraught when instead of agreeing to marry, her boyfriend ended their relationship. A fellow congregation member urged her to tell her parents, as it was now a problem of her whole family. Upon hearing the news, her father summoned Alva's boyfriend and his mother. Alva's boyfriend denied his paternity and his mother backed him up. They left the house without any agreement about the young man's responsibility in Alva's situation. That night, Alva's father was so upset by the unfolding events that he got into a fight with Alva and ended up beating her unconscious. After the fight her family took her to the hospital to recover. Alva lost the baby and perhaps faced permanent disability. While this example is extreme, reports of family violence directed toward young, unmarried pregnant women were fairly usual in my interviews. Family violence undoubtedly puts the mother and baby at direct health risk as well as increasing both maternal and fetal stress.

The stigma associated with these young, unmarried, pregnant women had mixed results in terms of their access to biomedical care during birth. Just as a young, married woman was locked into a social trajectory that coalesced around her birthing, a young, unmarried, pregnant woman was frequently locked out of such a trajectory. This freed her to go to the hospital during birth. Vilma's story was similar to several I heard. She was a high school student who hoped to finish her education, but got pregnant by mistake. Because her pregnancy was stigmatized and her father was ashamed, neither she nor he ever contacted a midwife about her condition. When it came time for her to give birth, her father took her to the hospital and left her there. Several days later, after she had given birth, he went and brought her home. During the weeks that I was in the emergency room I saw a number of teenagers walk in with their cousins or friends and give birth in the hospital.

But the stigma associated with illegitimate births can also work against a woman having access to biomedical care, as we saw with Mercedes, the young women who birthed alone. This point was recapitulated for me when Yovani came to my house one afternoon to deliver a message from his wife. With that business finished he asked me how dangerous it was for a woman to give birth if the baby is transverse across her stomach, instead of head down toward her pelvis. I asked him what was wrong, and he said that he was afraid because his younger sister had gotten pregnant and the baby had no father. She went alone to the health post one day to see the nurse and get free prenatal care. The nurse said that she was far along in her pregnancy, but that the baby was lying down across her stomach. The nurse told her that she would need a C-section or would likely die in labor. When his sister told the family what the nurse had said, his mother and father told her that she was not going anywhere but home to have that baby. She had gotten herself pregnant, and now she was going to have to deal with the consequences. No one was going to support her in helping her get to the hospital when her time came. They would not give her the money. They would not find transport for her. They would not go with her. Essentially, she had little choice but to follow her parents' wishes.

In sum, while marital status does seem to correlate with access to resources as the WHO predicts, it goes further to modulate pregnancy and birth risk in particular ways. Taking account of age, parity, and marital status together would create a better understanding of the kind of risk that unmarried pregnancy created in Sololá. While an older woman, who heads a household, might suffer most from a lack of monetary resources, a younger woman with no husband who finds herself pregnant might be at a real risk for violence. Her

situation also means that her access to biomedical care is less flexible: she either gets dropped off at the hospital, or is forbidden from
going.

Midwives and Birthing in the Village

As I argued in the last section, solidifying kin ties is an important
aspect of birthing in Santa Cruz. Yet just as important to a successful
birth is the involvement of an *iyom* (midwife). I begin this section
by exploring the characteristics of the iyom. While the campaign for
Safe Motherhood in Sololá tended to view the iyom as a practitioner of traditional medicine at best and a charlatan at worst, both of
these interpretations emphasize the focus on her ability to amelio-
rate physiological pathologies. Conceptualizing the iyom as a stand-
in biomedical practitioner, however, obscures the centrality of her
spiritual connections, which is perhaps her most important characteristic for her clients. My experience in Santa Cruz suggests that
both the practices of iyoma and the source of supernatural powers
that iyoma can tap into have changed with sweeping changes in
religious beliefs. These transformations are very important, because
they show how iyoma continue to be heavily imbricated in the social fabric of the village despite changes that would seem to preclude
this. Being delivered by a particular iyom solidifies integration into
religious communities.

Iyoma as Spiritual Providers

Within the framework of the WHO, midwives in Sololá are unskilled, traditional birth attendants, who have no biomedical training. So how does one become a midwife? The following story that
circulated during my fieldwork is fairly typical: a relatively wealthy
K'iche' family that lived a few villages above Santa Cruz had a teenage daughter who they were educating in Sololá, the capital of the
department. Being "modern" parents they hoped that their daughter would become a professional. She was a good student and was
apparently going to easily graduate from high school when an illness struck her. The parents began their search for a cure in the
hospital and offices of private doctors. When no one could find anything wrong with her, they took her to specialists. After exhausting
biomedical resources, they then began to visit herbalists, who examined the daughter and prescribed many treatments, but, again, none
worked. Finally, they visited a shaman. The shaman recognized that

the girl was being tortured because she was ignoring her "gift" to become a midwife. Instead of answering her calling, she was going to high school and preparing for a professional career. The parents eventually struck a bargain with the shaman. They would pay him a certain amount of money every month, which he would use to appease the spirit world, hopefully buying their daughter enough time to finish high school. After that they all agreed that she would have to become a midwife and follow her destiny, lest she live her whole life sick and incapacitated.

As this story so well points out, in this area of Sololá midwifery is a destiny, not a vocation (Paul 1975; Paul and Paul 1975). Women receive messages that reveal their calling. For example, in my own fieldwork, people reported incidents like being born with the amniotic sac intact as a sign of destiny.[13] Many others, like the Kaqchikel midwives who Linda V. Walsh (2006) interviewed, reported that dreams were an important sign. While interpreting theses signs may be difficult, their meaning becomes clear when a woman falls ill. The only way that she is able to overcome her illness is to begin to deliver babies. Up to this point, the iyom's story is clear.

Yet what is less clear is perhaps the iyom's most important credential: her "supernatural" powers. Lois Paul (1975:449–450) calls iyoma "sacred professionals" who, "like shamans ... owe their office to divine mandate, [whose] work is guided by supernatural tutelaries, and [whose] duties include ritual performances." The divine qualifications of iyoma in Sololá are referred to over and over again (Walsh 2006; Cosminsky 1977a; Cosminsky 1977b; Cosminsky 1982; Paul and Paul 1975). Walsh (2006:153) reads this continuity as supporting the idea that "in a span of more than 50 years ... spiritual beliefs and practices surrounding childbirth have remained constant among traditional healers." Yet how could spiritual beliefs and practices in the domain of childbirth remain constant when spiritual beliefs and practices at the village level have transformed so wildly over the last fifty years?

While Guatemala used to be a predominantly Catholic country, the conversion to Protestantism has now reached over 30 percent (Garrard-Burnett 2008). Changes in the religious landscape of Santa Cruz, where the vast majority of people are Evangelical, have reconfigured the iyom. She used to be a syncretic figure whose supernatural powers came from a variety of sources. Paul (1975:455) describes an *iyom's* parents performing ceremonies to protect her both at the Catholic Church and then sneaking out at night to "visit native shrines on the outskirts of the village, where the shaman of-

fered candles ... to the spirits ... and to the lords of many domains
of nature and calendric time."[14] This iyom, then, would have drawn
her power from the Catholic god, native Mayan gods, ancestral spirits, natural spirits, and those from her own day/name (on the Mayan calendar) group.[15] Yet, in the twenty-first century the change
in religion has reconfigured the power available for healers. Evangelicals only rely on the power of God, which is viewed as a good
(holy) power.

In Santa Cruz, where three of the five practicing midwives were
evangelical,[16] the spiritist roots of midwifery were being erased. Earlier descriptions of iyoma emphasize their ability to draw on the
entire spiritual world, which consists of both good and bad powers, to get a job done. Cruceños still believe in and attribute agency
to this spirit world. Nevertheless, they say, a real devout Christian
would never appeal to any power other than the Christian God.
And indeed, in interviews and in conversations with iyoma, women
continually stressed that the power of the iyom lay in her connection to the Christian God, not in her ability to call on spirits or her
knowledge of herbs and medicine. The iyom, I heard over and over
again, was there to do God's bidding; she finished what God started
when He made a new life in a woman's belly. The connection between God's direction and the practice of midwifery was also emphasized by iyoma themselves, who claimed they relied on divine
intervention to guide their actions when attending a birth. During
interviews and informal conversations, no midwife or woman ever
referred to calling on spiritual powers other than God's to help with
a pregnancy-related problem.

It is quite impressive that midwives in Santa Cruz have been able
to weather this profound religious change, given that shamans were
not. The inherent conflict between shamanism and evangelism was
drawn to the fore publicly in Santa Cruz during the 1980s. As Lisa
Anne Schaumann (1993) relates, the village's last shaman was convinced to "retire" by his son, who had converted to evangelism, became a pastor, and was trying to save his father from hell. After
years of speaking out against him, he finally convinced his father
to mend his ways and stop his sinful practice (i.e., speaking to the
spirit world). Iyoma have been able to survive, however, by paring
down their practice; while midwives worldwide are commonly described as the bearers of traditional medicine, skilled in the use of
herbs for everything from abortifacients to curtailing hemorrhages
(Jolly 2002), Cruceña iyoma are most identified for the power of
their prayer. Women who narrated stories of their birthing difficul-

ties often described to me in detail that after a problem was identified they would get on their knees with their midwives and pray for their birth to get back on track.[17]

A Midwife's Job is to Deliver Babies

As I worked in Sololá with the iyoma, studied the policies laid out by the Safe Motherhood campaign, and sat in on training sessions involving health workers and iyoma, I realized that a good understanding of the iyom's role was lacking. Iyoma were basically treated as if they were unskilled biomedical obstetricians, and there was an assumption that they would function within the system the same as an unskilled health worker might. Since both iyoma and obstetricians are called upon to ensure that a birth goes well, health workers just assumed that their roles were roughly the same. Yet, while the activities of an obstetrician and an iyom might intersect, there were also very important differences; unlike the obstetrician, an iyom was not valued for her knowledge or treatment of pathologies, but for the powers that she derived from God. When something went wrong in the village and a birthing woman died, the knowledge of the midwife was not instantly brought into question. As many women I interviewed repeated over and over, the midwife is only there to do her work, which is to deliver the baby. She is carrying out God's will and is only there to help. How could any problems in the birth be associated with her? In fact, as the story below illustrates, pathologies fell outside of the realm of her expertise.

During my first year of fieldwork in Santa Cruz I was sitting with my husband in a little office that I had set up next to the health post in the central square. At about 10:00 AM a man whom I didn't know came to the door. Addressing us in Spanish he said that they needed some advice, because there was a woman giving birth and she wasn't talking anymore. My husband asked the woman's name. The man said that he didn't know, but he could show us where she lived. As the nurse was gone and there were no other biomedical personnel in the village, I again grabbed the book *Where Women Have No Doctor,* and we headed to the house.

As we approached I saw a group of children from teens to toddlers filling the courtyard between two one-room adobe houses. Some were obviously waiting for news about their mother or aunt, while others had shown up for the spectacle itself and were playing, waiting for something to happen. We traversed a treacherous mud path that lead down a steep slope and when we got to one of the adobe houses, the man signaled for us to go in. Woven cloth had been affixed to the wooden frame of the only window in the room, and as a result it was both dark and hot inside. The air was pungent with the odor of herbs, and the room was filled to the brim with adults, several of whom were wailing. Despite the darkness it was not difficult to identify Geronima, who was lying on the floor on a pile of cloth. Her husband had her torso propped up on his legs, and his arms were under hers supporting her. She was in her huipil and *corte*[18] and was covered with blankets. As my eyes accustomed to the dark I identified Nersa, an elderly woman and one of six midwives in the village, and asked her in Kaqchikel what had happened. She told me that the family had told her that Geronima was complaining about a strong headache at 8:00 PM the night before. Suddenly, she cried out that she saw a bad spirit and then she collapsed immediately. Geronima's husband had not called Nersa until 8:00 AM the next morning.

One of Geronima's family members broke in and said that Geronima was stiff and had been shaking. Nersa concurred. She insisted that I feel where the baby was. Reluctantly, I washed my hands in the water that was sitting in a receptacle next to Geronima, stuck my hand under her corte and began to put two fingers inside of her vagina. I instantly butted up against the head of the baby, which was probably one or two inches inside her. Trying to assess the situation, I asked Nersa several times if she thought Geronima was strong enough to have the baby. She responded several times that Geronima was sick, and that it was not the pregnancy, but the sickness that was stopping her from having the baby. I felt helpless, confused, and frustrated that Nersa would not directly answer the question. Was Geronima going to have the baby or was it stuck?

Considering the station of the baby's head and the fact that this was Geronima's twelfth gestation, Geronima's family decided to wait one more hour before leaving to find help. My husband would go make a stretcher and find some men to help carry her. I would stay with Geronima and her family. If the baby was not born within that hour we would go to the hospital.

At 10:40 AM my husband left and the rest of us waited. One of the wailing women, who was Geronima's sister, kept telling Nersa to do something. Nersa took a piece of a dry herb and gave it to someone, who crushed it in their hands and rubbed it under Geronima's nose. Judging by the amount of residue that covered her face and huipil, this act had been repeated numerous times already. Nersa then washed her hands with a bar of soap in the same receptacle of water that I had used, dried them on her apron, squirted oil from an old water bottle onto her hands, reached under Geronima's huipil, and massaged her belly. Then we waited. I started timing Geronima's contractions, watching her face and her body for signs of her muscles working. Geronima indeed was not talking and it was hard to tell if she was conscious or not, which made the situation all the more confusing. About twenty minutes after I had been sitting there, Geronima began to convulse: her entire body tensed and she thrashed around. The seizure lasted for about half a minute, and afterward the wailing began more intensely than before. I was terrified. Nersa immediately felt the baby again and said that it had receded. She looked at me and said that what I just saw was the sickness. It was the problem. It was just pushing the baby back into the mother.

The only thing that I knew how to do at that point was to go to the hospital. I started to negotiate with her husband, who was in agreement that we go. Both of Geronima's sisters protested that if we took her to the hospital she would die. Nersa was ambivalent; she agreed that the sickness was bad, but was afraid that Geronima would need to give birth in the street before we got to the hospital. Geronima convulsed again, and her sisters asked Nersa to massage her. Once more Nersa washed her hands in the same receptacle of water, covered her hands with oil that she squirted out of the water bottle, and started to massage Geronima's belly again.

At about 11:20 AM my husband returned with a cloth stretched between two poles and four men to help him carry. After some negotiating Geronima was on the stretcher, covered from head to toe with blankets, and being carried on a ten-minute walk down the mountain to the dock to catch a boat where an ambulance would be waiting. As the group made its way down the mountainside, it turned into an extensive entourage. When we got to the boat the men tried to position the stretcher over the benches, but while the poles lay nicely across them, Geronima's body sagged in the gaps in between. Nersa enlisted me in trying to hold her legs apart, which was incredibly difficult. Halfway through the boat journey I looked under the blanket and saw a baby nestled into the space between Geronima's legs, completely out of the mother. He had a full head of hair and was perfectly shaped. He looked beautiful. I couldn't figure out why Nersa wasn't doing anything with him. One of the stretcher holders, who was right behind me, kept telling me to pick the baby up and try to save him, so I interrupted Nersa and asked her about the baby. She looked at me and shook her head, at which point I realized that the baby had been born dead.

Eventually, we got to the hospital where my husband and Geronima's husband accompanied her into the ER, and the rest of us sat outside on the benches, only catching glimpses of what was going on when the door swung open and closed. Nersa insisted that I go in and tell the doctor that the placenta had not yet come out. I went into the ER to tell them, and the doctor told me not to worry since it had come out when we arrived. After a few minutes Geronima's husband emerged from the ER, as there was nothing more he could do. Some family members asked him about the baby. The baby was dead, he told us, but he didn't know what would happen to the body. He said that Geronima was going to have to stay in the hospital. Several of the people who accompanied us then became concerned. They insisted I go back into the ER and make sure that no one confused Geronima with someone else. They told me that so often when you stay in the hospital things happen: the staff don't know what treatment you had already received, or they confuse you with someone else, and then you ended up getting killed because they gave you something bad or the same medicine twice. I went back in again and explained the fears to my husband, who talked to the doctor. The doctor promised that no one was going to confuse Geronima with another patient and assured us that she herself would be on call all night and would watch over Geronima. I reported the doctor's words to Geronima's family.

As there was nothing else anyone could do, we all left the hospital. It was around 2:00 PM by the time we got home—four hours since the man had come to ask our help.

Since this tragedy happened only a few months into my fieldwork, I had not developed the relationships that exposed me to the minutiae of handling an event like this in a village like Santa Cruz. Evacuating Geronima did not bind me to her family. After taking her to the hospital I relied on others to bring me the news of what happened.

I hoped that taking Geronima to the hospital would save her and looked forward to hearing my husband's report when he returned from the hospital the next day.[19] But when he got home that evening he told me that Geronima's organs had begun to fail during the night. The doctor on call had requested that they send her to the central hospital in Guatemala City that was better equipped to deal with cases like hers. Much to the doctor's chagrin, Geronima's husband, however, had refused the transfer.[20] Two days after we had taken her to the hospital, we heard over the loudspeaker in the village that Geronima's family would shortly arrive at the dock with her body.

The tragedy of Geronima's death did not end that day. Her return to the village was as dramatic as her departure had been. Publicly, I participated in the rituals associated with her death: her body sailed back to the village in a casket, the family held a wake, and the next day she was transported to the cemetery to be buried. Perhaps a week or two after her body was returned to the village I noticed a man passed out in the central square as I arrived to the health post in the morning. When I asked, neighbors told me that it was Geronima's husband. Since the death he had begun to drink to numb his own grief. This left his young teenage daughter to step in and take her mother's place. Several months later Geronima's youngest child, a 3 year old, died. Without a mother or father to look after him, he didn't stand a chance.

A week after Geronima's body returned, a representative of the Guatemalan Ministry of Health arrived to discuss her death with the village midwives. She had died, he said, of eclampsia. High blood pressure associated with Geronima's eclampsia caused her to see stars and lights dancing in her vision, which she mistook for spirits visiting her. The toxemia of her pregnancy was by then far too much for her body to handle, so she fainted. As she received no medical help her condition worsened and she began to convulse. The convulsions contributed to the extended birthing time and acute fetal stress, which killed the baby. As there was little that the local hospital could do for someone in such a critical condition, she died of massive organ failure. While it was quite sad that Geronima had died, in the official eyes, there was nothing that the midwife could have done to help her.

After the meeting I compared the Ministry's explanation of Geronima's death with Nersa's.[21] When I had arrived to Geronima's house, the first thing that Nersa did was emphasize that Geronima's problem was not related to her birth, but rather her sickness. For Nersa, all of the elements of a normal birth were there: Geronima was over nine months pregnant; she was fully dilated, and she was having consistent contractions that were pushing the baby out. It was the sickness that happened to present itself at the same time as the birth that was complicating the matter. Geronima's husband also concurred with the separation of the sickness from the birth. Even though Geronima, who was full term, had collapsed at 8:00 PM the previous night, no one sought out the help of the iyom until the next morning, when it became obvious that Geronima was in labor.

Nersa's interpretation of Geronima's woes was decidedly different from those offered by the Ministry of Health doctor. While the

doctor's explanations of why Geronima's birth went awry emphasize physiological dysfunction that affected her body, Nersa's narrative concentrates on the fact that Geronima saw spirits, and that
the spirits were probably causing her sickness. Though the sickness,
most readily represented in Geronima's convulsions, was temporally
concurrent with her labor, in describing to me what was happening
Nersa separated the two by emphasizing that the birth was normal
but the sickness was hampering the birth's progress. Indeed, the focus on the sickness foreshadowed the maelstrom that ensued after
Geronima's death. Why had she seen spirits? Was someone cursing
her? Her husband? Her midwife?

The interpretation of Geronima's death concurred in important
ways with the interpretation of Rosario's death that began this book.
Geronima undoubtedly experienced physical problems that ultimately
led to her death, these physical problems were viewed conclusively
as symptoms of a *social* breakdown—the broken relationship with an
unknown party. This social breakdown resulted in her being cursed,
as evidenced by her encounter with malevolent spirits.

As this example demonstrates, the iyom's role is as more of a
spiritual conduit than a biomedical intervener. Indeed, the current
widespread co-option of the Spanish evangelical term *testiga* (witness)[22] into Kaqchikel to refer to the midwife summarizes well her
role. The midwife is there to witness God's work. She is also God's
agent to help along the birth. Her main attraction or skill is not her
ability to identify or handle pathologies.

The idea that there is a difference between the iyom, who delivers babies, and the obstetrician, who delivers babies and handles
pathologies, was further underscored during my time in the emergency room in the Sololá hospital. I found it very perplexing that
of the sixty-four obstetric cases that I observed enter the ER, iyoma
only accompanied fourteen women. Why weren't the iyoma coming
to the ER? I had been present during meetings when health workers
had told the midwives that they should never abandon their clients
and that they should always come to the ER. Were the iyoma irresponsible? Were they afraid of what the doctors might say to them?
When interviewing in the hospital I asked families and later the
women themselves if they had contacted the midwife before coming
to the hospital. But people told me that they never contacted their
midwife if they had a pre-term miscarriage. Nor were the iyoma
ever present for post-partum complications, such as an infection.
Indeed, save one case, midwives only accompanied women when
problems appeared during labor—i.e., obstructions, pre-eclampsia,

prolonged labor, etc.[23] What I found in the hospital only further helps conceptually define the iyom—her main job is to deliver babies and she receives guidance from God to do just that. This clarification of the role of the midwife as an individual who has a special gift for delivering babies, rather than as a specialist of all pregnancy-related difficulties, further shows how the domains of a biomedical attendant and iyom may overlap but are not coterminous. Though midwives are interested and eclectic in their approaches to birth, frequently incorporating new biomedical knowledge into their practice, it would be a mistake to narrowly conceive of them as biomedical "wanna-bes." Accordingly, their identification of pregnancy "problems" is undoubtedly influenced by divergent practices and the divergent meanings assigned to birthing events.

The Safe Motherhood campaign in Sololá, however, failed to distinguish between the responsibilities and roles of an iyom and those of a biomedical worker. The monthly meetings that the Ministry of Health held with the iyoma frequently began by reviewing stories of maternal deaths that occurred since the last meeting. The major guidelines concerning how to identify pathology and when to refer a client were always refreshed. But the stories would also contain an undertone of judging if the iyom involved in the birth had acted appropriately or not. For example, one such meeting of midwives and health workers began by describing the recent death of a woman from Chichicastenango. The woman was 35 and had four children at home. When she went into labor her husband called the midwife. The midwife came and delivered the baby without problems but the placenta never came out. One hour passed. Two hours passed and still no placenta. The family asked if everything was okay. The midwife told them not to worry, that the placenta would still come. Three hours passed. Four hours passed. Finally, six hours after the baby had been birthed, the midwife said that she thought that there was a problem. The family then went to look for transport. It took time to find an available car and drive the woman to the hospital, and eight hours after the birth she finally arrived. Unfortunately, the woman had lost too much blood in the intervening time and died. The Ministry of Health guideline is that if the placenta does not come out within half an hour of the birth, the midwife should get the woman to a hospital immediately. In this example, we were told, the midwife was at fault because she delayed the transfer of the woman for too long.

While a biomedical health worker would undoubtedly be guilty for delaying a referral, it is not so clear that this onus transfers to the iyom. During my interviews I asked women if they thought that a woman who had died from a problem related to her pregnancy or birth could have been saved if she had sought medical care in the hospital. Almost resoundingly, the answer was affirmative. But when I asked who is to blame when a woman dies from a pregnancy or birthing-related problem, most women said that the woman's own fate is the central cause of her death.[24] When I then pressed the issue and asked if a women ever died because the midwife did not seek help quickly enough, very few women viewed the actions of the midwife as implicated in the death of her client. The midwife, they stressed, is there to help. It is not her fault if something goes wrong with the birth.

The differences between what the biomedical providers expected of the iyom and what her clients wanted were only concretized for me when Neli, a midwife from another village, brought a young woman with a transverse pregnancy to the emergency room. Neli was one of the younger iyoma, was literate, and intellectually certainly understood the Ministry of Health recommendation that no transverse pregnancy be delivered at home. Nevertheless, Neli had tried to attend to the young woman. I wasn't at the hospital when a health worker berated her,[25] but I talked to Neli after the fact. She told me that the young woman's parents-in-law were very adamant that the baby be born at home, despite the fact that Neli had told them that she didn't think that it was possible. Nevertheless, it was Neli's responsibility to serve her community, and if a young woman was in the throes of birth, she could not abandon that girl. According to her own logic, it would be selfish for Neli to withhold her gift from someone who needed it.

This examples helps illustrate two crucial points. The first is that the authority of the iyom and the biomedical provider are widely different. The Safe Motherhood campaign imagines that what happens in a biomedical setting happens in the village; as soon as an iyom comes onto the scene the care of a birthing woman passes onto her, and she then calls the shots. Yet iyoma are first and foremost servants to their communities. They have an obligation to God, who has given them the power to deliver babies, and to their neighbors to help. Ultimately, they do not have the authority to obligate anyone to do anything.[26] The second point is that the Ministry of Health may be shooting itself in the foot by assuming that midwives are to blame. As Servando Hinojosa (2004) points out, the Ministry of Health in Guatemala is dependent on midwives to have access to pregnant and birthing women. Yet it is sabotaging itself by assuming

that midwives will behave in ways that step outside of the bounds
of their roles as spiritual providers, and then becoming upset when
iyoma don't. For her part, Neli was quite unhappy about how she
was treated when she finally arrived to the hospital with the young
woman. The health workers had doubts about the future of their
campaign, and Neli was probably equally skeptical about continuing
to cooperate with them.

While women relied on the iyoma, they also acknowledged that
if you have a lot of pain and your birth is so problematic that the
midwife can't help you any more, you have little choice but to go to
the hospital. It was the logical next step. A number of women who
I interviewed said that they themselves had gone to the hospital at
some point or another for obstetric care. Yet many also said that they
would exhaust all other resources before turning to the hospital. To
understand why this might be, in the next chapter I look at what happens to a woman who goes to the ER with an obstetric emergency.

Intervening in Birth and Women's Agency

A detailed look at birth in Santa Cruz helps highlight the crucial
connection between biological events and social worlds. Thinking
of the connection in relation to biosocial subjectivities pushes us
beyond merely noting how the biological and social correspond, to
instead examine biological processes as constitutive of individual
understandings of the social and vice versa. In Santa Cruz the physical birthing event serves as a real-time enactment of each family
member's place in the world. For a young married woman birth also
does something[27]—it integrates the couple and binds them into a
larger family unit. As we saw in the story of Lisbeth, who had been
abandoned by her husband, birth remained a crucial site for Lisbeth's in-laws to (re)affirm their interdependence as a family. As
I argued in the introduction, the events described in this chapter
both portray and reinstantiate an understanding of one's place in
the world as intimately connected to others.

Yet the value of birthing at home was not solely predicated on the
ability of the family to be together (which was not allowed at hospital births). For strengthening the connection between a woman and
her in-laws, birthing at the in-laws' home, as opposed to another
location, was symbolic. Birthing at home also allowed the important
participation of the midwife. Each midwife was chosen and revered
not because of her skill in dealing with an emergency, but because

of her legitimacy in the eyes of God. As a spiritual provider, the midwife helped integrate a pregnancy and birth into the wider religious community. Her absence from the process was equally as suspect in shedding moral doubt on a pregnancy. These additional factors anchored kin to particular places in Santa Cruz (e.g., a specific compound or church), and formed part of their understanding of their own subjectivity.

In my analysis these everyday interactions are paramount to the construction of a relational subjectivity, and therefore, an initiative to curb maternal mortality that changes the birthing event threatens this subjectivity. I am not arguing that pregnancy and birth are the only places where subjectivities are produced in real-time interactions. Rather, because pregnancy and birth are two sites where biological and social meet, they should be understood as privileged sites to construct subjectivities. Pregnancy and birth provide significant opportunities to transform the social world by transforming webs of relations. For relational subjects, this inevitably means a change in the understanding of one's place in the world. I argue that the erasure of these sites is, therefore, not trivial. Any event that weakens—whether intentionally or not—the social fabric of kinship in a poor community that depends on reciprocity to survive should not be read as inconsequential.[28]

The danger of this position is that it be misread as a romantic attachment to traditionalism or, even worse, as an endorsement of gender oppression. I would reject either of these assertions. My point in highlighting the potential effects of the Safe Motherhood campaign to work as a vehicle that disenfranchises indigenous Kaqchikel villagers in Santa Cruz of their patrimony is not to reject change writ large.[29] Rather, it is a plea for a more nuanced and comprehensive evaluation of the effects of development projects. Development projects inevitably have unintended consequences that spread into wider social life.[30] These unintended consequences need to be examined so that decisions to promote change, such as the transformation of subjectivity in a Kaqchikel village, are conscious ones, rather than an invisible side effect. The system of birth that I have described is also arguably patriarchal, in the sense that it is predicated on the dominance of a male father of the family.[31] Subordination is expected along both age and gendered lines, so that young women who move in with their affines are expected to be obedient to both their husbands and in-laws. A knee-jerk feminist call for eradication of such a system unintentionally "rationalizes the planned management and liberation of women in the South by Westernized professionals in the development apparatus" (Saunders 2002:14), creating a moral cover that lionizes middle-class western women while potentially having deleterious effects on women's health. For example, B. C. Mullany, M. J. Hindin, and S. Becker (2005) demonstrate how development programs aiming to empower women and make them more autonomous can impede men's (continued) participation in caring for a woman's pregnancy. In short, a feminist agenda is more complex than merely identifying and condemning gender-based inequality.

The scholars that I have drawn on to help me understand relational subjectivities, Marilyn Strathern and Suad Joseph, both use the concept to theorize women's subordination. Strathern (1988) explored relational selves in Melanesia to expose the incommensurability of western academic units of analysis, more specifically by showing the limits of western feminism in the Melanesian context. She employed the concept of relational selves to de-center our (universal) understanding of gender hierarchy. Her example served as a critique of western feminist inclinations to center our understanding of gender in the universal oppression of women by men. As she (28) explains it, "ethnographic accounts of other societies cannot be seen [by feminists] as simply a more or less unbiased elucidation on the subordination or freedom of women." Such a tendency missed that ideologies of gender subordination are particular and closely connected to social life.

Joseph's (1994) ethnographic account illustrates particularly well how gender subordination is closely connected to social life. Joseph uses the concept of connectivity to trace the psychodynamic processes through which gender and hierarchy are learned and reinstantiated. She argues that the brother and sister relationship is the proving ground of Arab patriarchy. The relationship is characterized by "love/nurturance and power/violence" dynamics in which "[y]oung females learned feminine roles by submitting to brothers. Young males learned to be a patriarch by practicing first on their sisters and younger brothers" (66). Only by understanding the ethnographic particulars can we begin to understand modes through which young women and men are subordinated, and how they exercise power. For example, brothers and sisters could "use their relationship ... to contest their fathers' authority" (66). The connectivity between a sister and brother also meant that a sister could motivate her brother into action through her own actions.

A focus on subordination in the example of birth and pregnancy that I present here similarly impoverishes our understanding of

women's lives and agency in these households. As Sumi Madhok
(2004) maintains, when women live in contexts where they are subordinated, we need to amplify our understanding of agency to include examples of inaction as well as action. Applying this example,
we need to consider women's participation in homebirth as women
exercising their agency, not just being subordinated. To make her
case Madhok (225) argues that "autonomy ... focuses on the ability
of persons to engage with moral ideas and to introduce a change in
their moral repertoire subsequent to these engagements." She illustrates her argument through examples of women who express preferences antithetical to those of mothers-in-law or husbands who
oppress them. Not all women are able to act on their preference, so
it is the formation of preference that constitutes agency for Madhok. In her own piece she can only identify agency in disconnects
between preferences (of mothers-in-law and daughters-in-law, for
example). Yet the "ability of persons to engage with moral ideas" or
to change those moral ideas is not necessarily defined by resistance.
In other words, agency is not defined by resistance (Abu-Lughod
1990). It may also be defined by actively seeking to form alliance or
cooperate or any other activity that does not involve conflict.

I would argue that women's decision to birth at home is, in most
cases, not one imposed on them, but rather should be understood
as a preference. The birth experience is such that labor pains frequently preclude a woman's ability to care for herself or tempers
her interest in making a decision. This is precisely the time when
someone wants to feel accompanied,[32] and preferably cared for. A
woman who births at home with her husband and family surrounding her knows that she will be emotionally and physically cared for.
Just as she shows respect to her in-laws by, for example, using the
midwife her mother-in-law suggests, her in-laws will be responsible
for guarding her health during birth. While a woman gestated a
baby over many months and must push it out, her husband must
support her during the labor—he will physically hold her up. The
birth is a family performance. While it is simple to see hierarchy in
almost any of the stories I present here around pregnancy and birth,
it is difficult to imagine that a woman would prefer to undertake
it on her own. Yet that is precisely what the choice to birth in the
hospital would represent. In these terms, then, I find homebirth an
explicit exercise of women's agency—women prefer to and do stay
home. This preference speaks to the importance of kin ties in *supporting* women, as well as in subordinating them.

Chapter 2

COMING TO THE ER

ANALYSIS OF AN INTERACTION

After I had observed about thirty obstetric emergencies enter the ER, I felt like I had a good enough idea of what was going on to start doing audio recordings. But before I could record I had to figure out how to set up my equipment. I brought the rather long microphone and the minidisc recorder that I would use and enlisted the help of the doctors, nurses, and others to create a setup. How and where would I suspend my mic? It needed to be placed somewhere inconspicuous, yet easy for me to reach. The more centrally located, the more voices it would pick up. Yet it couldn't be on any surface that could move, like the beds or tables, because that would create too much feedback. The walls were solid concrete, and it would be difficult to attach anything to them. I thought that maybe I could stand on a chair or one of the beds and suspend the microphone from the ceiling, which was very high, but no one relished the idea of me climbing up and down and balancing dangerously to get the mic. Finally, one of the staff came back with a coat hanger and some pliers, and he quickly bent it to make a mic stand that I could slip between the window and its metal frame. It was easy to reach, easy to set up, and allowed me to leave the minidisc player inconspicuously on the window sill. I started recording and we all walked around the room, talking from different points, trying to figure out where on the window I should hang the mic to get the best coverage of the room.

While everyone easily understood what it was that I was doing—i.e., recording women who came in with obstetric emergencies—

they didn't necessarily understand why. As I sketched out in the introduction, making recordings was important to me for several reasons. My work is predicated on those of scholars who view interactions and linguistic practices as an important site for studying what actually might be going on between institutions and their clients (Menéndez 1990; Drew 1992; Silverman 1997; McDermott and Tylbor 1995). Everyday interactions can index power relations between social classes (Bernstein 1975; Labov 1972), genders (Tannen 1993), status (Brown and Levinson 1987), or ethnicities (Woolard 1985). By looking at interactions we can understand the strategies that social actors use to accomplish tasks—for example, what exactly do clients do to collaborate, collude, or contest treatment that they dislike at the hospital? Why would they choose the strategies that they do? Are other strategies open to them? Recordings allowed me access to a much more detailed and faithful reproduction of interactions than any other method I used. I could replay them over and over. I could go back and look for small details that I might not have noticed before.

This chapter is based on a transcript that I made of the interactions surrounding the arrival of a woman named Guadalupe to the hospital to receive emergency obstetric care. While her birth went well, her family brought her to the hospital because her placenta failed to come out. The recording concerns interactions between the nurse and the family. The nurse misled Guadalupe's family about why Guadalupe had to stay at the hospital; she needed antibiotics to prevent infection, but the nurse insinuated that she needed to stay because Guadalupe's vagina was damaged during the birth.

The crux of this chapter is to investigate the reasons the nurse would have to mislead the family. Rather than framing the nurse's behavior as idiosyncratic, I instead highlight how Guadalupe's experience is better explained with reference to a system that actively promotes the biologization and medicalization of birth.[1] I read the nurse's lie as an attempt to convince the family that Guadalupe did not receive good care in Chupöl, her native village, and why it was of utmost importance that they let Guadalupe stay in the hospital. Throughout the interaction the nurse was trying to make the strongest case possible for why this family should not rely on midwives and homebirth. She wanted to undermine the family's faith that they could get good help if they were to take Guadalupe home. She was attempting to convert them into trusting users of the hospital through juxtaposing the competence of biomedical care with the incompetence of "traditional" care. Her message was that Guadalupe's family needed to accept and correctly use "modern" biomedical care.

I begin this chapter with a brief description of the layout of the hospital. I then turn to Guadalupe's own background and follow this with a verbatim description of what was said in the emergency room.[2] Presenting such a detailed account of the interaction will certainly help clarify precisely what makes these visits to the hospital so daunting for poor, Mayan families.

Seeking Emergency Obstetric Help in the Hospital

There was only one opening in the concrete wall that surrounded the hospital and the first obstacle to be traversed upon arriving was to get through this gate. The small gatehouse, which was directly inside of the wall, was manned twenty-four hours a day and was the main communication post with the outside world; all incoming telephone calls and arriving patients and visitors had to go through it.[3]

After traversing the gate the next step was to get into the emergency room. The words were clearly marked on a pair of double glass doors leading into the hospital building. Through the doors was an antechamber, which served as the nexus of two hallways, a few wooden benches lined the walls and there was an opaque door next to one of the benches. Coming from the US where there are sign posts, directions, and information booths, I found arriving to the ER disorienting since there was no one there to greet you or tell you what to do next. In fact, the first time I went there it was difficult for me to tell if we were supposed to continue walking down one of the halls, knock on the opaque door, or just sit down.[4]

Going through the opaque door, you entered the emergency room itself. To your left was a large metal desk with a pressed wood top. The desk had a phone and a small pile of forms, but was essentially available to anyone as a work space. Next to the desk was a Health-o-meter scale, and next to that was a wood cabinet for storing drugs. The knobs had been replaced with metal eyebolts. The top section closed via a sliding bolt set into the wood, and the bottom section was secured with a padlock that fit through a hasp attached to one side and an eye on the other.

The room was divided into four different sick bays. Two of them had stationary beds with vinyl covered cushions that were taped with medical tape to a metal bed frame and the other two beds had full mattresses. The room could be bisected with long flower-print sheets suspended by shower rings on black metal rods. Each of the bed areas could be made private by pulling another curtain around the bed. The curtains were generally left open unless someone was changing, being attended to, or in very bad shape. The two bays on the opposite side of the room from the desk each had built-in concrete countertops beside the beds. The counters were covered with medical supplies. Old glass containers for instant coffee were filled with different cottons, pull-top water bottles were filled with different colored antiseptics and cleaning solutions. A metal cup was filled with hemostats and there was a test tube holder. A five-gallon bucket from Tim Horton's had been converted into a trash can and a small wooden foot stool to help patients climb up to the bed was shoved underneath.

In the back of the room was a wide door that separated obstetric patients from the others. The obstetric patients were treated in a room about a third of the size of the main room, which had two beds next to each other. The area was made more private by a curtain that separated the beds from the rest of the room. The hospital also had a moveable screen, which could be used to obscure the view of one obstetric patient from another. At the foot of the beds was a metal tray that served as a counter. Some medical supplies like cotton and antiseptic were on the tray. As part of the effort to improve emergency obstetric care, the procedures for treating several of the most common problems that doctors would encounter had been written on poster board, laminated, and hung on the wall to remind doctors of how to stop a hemorrhage or treat pre-eclampsia.

The comings and goings of the patients in the ER were basically controlled by one auxiliary nurse. She would keep a running mental record of who was outside, who was inside, whether or not a specialist had been called to see them, what they needed, what they had been given, where they were in their paperwork, etc. These nurses' ability to categorize and remember who was going through the ER was impressive. When the nurses changed shifts, the one going off had to debrief the one coming onto duty, telling her, among other things, who was in bed, who was in the bathroom, who was over in X-ray, and who was outside waiting for what. Through two months in the ER I never saw a patient forgotten.

Once the patient was ensconced in bed, a nurse assessed him/her to determine which doctor needed to be paged over the hospital-wide intercom system. While there was always an auxiliary nurse and a general practitioner (GP) working in the ER, Monday through Friday in the afternoons, four specialists, including an obstetrician/

gynecologist, were also present. While the GP was always on duty in the ER, during the afternoon the specialists had to make their rounds on the wards, as well as attend to ER patients.

After being paged the doctor would arrive, perform an exam, and decide treatment. He would talk to the family and complete a more in-depth medical history. If an obstetric patient was to be admitted she would then change into a hospital gown. If it seemed that a woman could not do it herself, her family was asked to come in and help.[5] Since all maternity patients had to enter the hospital through the obstetric ER, doctors would see a mix of healthy women in labor; women who needed to be prepped for scheduled c-sections; women who were referred by *consulta externa* (outpatient care) because of some pregnancy complication (like high blood pressure) who need to be interned; many pregnant women with urinary tract infections, who were normally not admitted; women with dead fetuses and miscarriages; and finally, a subset who had obstetric emergencies.

Doctors and nurses were inconsistent about whether or not a patient's family or her midwife could stay with her while she was being treated. For procedures that could be quite gory, such as manual extraction of the placenta, they usually asked family to leave. However, for other procedures, including vaginal exams, female family members were usually present. Sometimes family members wandered in and out and had to be asked several times to leave. Other times their itinerancy was tolerated.

Guadalupe's Trip to the Hospital

Guadalupe lived with her husband and in-laws in a *cantón* (rural community) near the city of Chichicastenango. Her in-laws felt that there was only one good midwife in their village and they contracted her to help with the birth of Guadalupe's first child. While the baby was born healthy, Guadalupe's placenta did not come out after the birth. After about half an hour the midwife decided that Guadalupe's placenta was stuck and she advised the family to go to the clinic. Since Guadalupe's in-laws did not trust the skill of any of the other midwives, everyone decided that it was best to bring Guadalupe to the hospital. After contracting her uncle to take them in the back of a pick-up, her husband and in-laws joined her on the one and a half hour journey to the Sololá hospital. The newborn was left behind with Guadalupe's mother who was charged with finding a wet nurse.

When they arrived at 12:18 PM one of the drivers went into the emergency room to get a stretcher, which he wheeled out to the pick-up truck so that they could transfer Guadalupe from the flat bed onto it. One minute later they had her in the ER. The nurse asked her husband to bring her back to the OB section of the ER, and to place her on the bed behind one of the curtains. She then asked everyone to leave. The two men who drove the truck left, but Guadalupe's husband stayed and her mother-in-law and father-in-law wandered in and out, bringing some things in and taking others away.

Enfermera: Venga, ayudarme a mí por favor. ... Cuantos niños tiene?
1 Nurse: Come help me please. ... How many children does she
2 have?

Esposo: La primera.
3 Husband: It's the first.

En. Es el primer bebe?
4 N: It's the first baby?

Es: Si, la primera.
5 H: Yes, the first.

E: Muy bien. ... Si pues ... Ciérrame la puerta allá, señor, por favor.
6 N: Okay. ... Well ... Close that door for me, sir, please.

Es: Muy bien. ... Cual? Este?
7 H: Okay. ... Which? This one?

[He closes the door from the antechamber of the obstetric ER to the hall, where the men are waiting.]

En: ¡Huy! Esta superpalida usted. ... Ha sangrado mucho? Ha sangrado mucho?
8 N: Oooh! You are incredibly pale. ... Did you bleed a lot? Did she
9 bleed a lot?

Es: No.
10 H: No.

En: O estaba muy pálida cuando estaba embarazada?
11 N: Or was she really pale when she was pregnant?

Es: Si estaba un poquito pálida.
12 H: Yes, she was a little pale.

[The nurse asks questions and they remove Guadalupe from the stretcher.]

En: Párese para allá, por favor. ... Arrastradito. ... Quien es el esposo de ella?
13 N: Please stand over there. ... Slide her. ... Who is her husband?

Es: Yo soy.
14 H: I am.

En: Vaya.
15 N: Okay.

Es: Esto lo sacamos afuera?
16 H: Should we take this [referring to the stretcher] outside?

En: Si por favor. ... Como se llama Usted?
17 N: Yes please. ... What is your name?

[The husband asks her in K'iche' and Guadalupe gives her full name.]

En: Baja la lengua. ... Cierra me la boca.
18 N: Stick out your tongue. ... Close your mouth for me.

[The nurse inserts a thermometer as Guadalupe's husband again translates what the nurse says.]

En: Si me hacen favor, todos se me esperan afuera, si necesito algo yo les llamo.
19 N: If you would all do me a favor and wait outside, if I need any-
20 thing, I'll call you.

Es: Vaya. Muy bien.
21 H: Sure. Okay.

[The nurse leaves to call the doctor over the intercom. Guadalupe's mother-in-law and husband stay with her, and the three continue to converse in whispers. At 12:25 PM the nurse checks on them.]

En: Ahorita va a venir el doctor, oye?
22 N: In a moment the doctor will come, do you hear?

Es: Vaya.
23 H: Sure.

[At 12:28 PM the nurse returns with hospital clothes for Guadalupe to wear.]

En: Quítate la ropa por favor.
24 N: Please take your clothes off.

Es: Muy bien.
25 H: Okay.

En: Quitase usted esto mire.
26 N: Take this off, look.

[The nurse demonstrates how to get Guadalupe's clothes off for her family.]

En: Solo déjalo así.
27 N: Just leave it like this.

[The family continues to try to arrange her clothes.]

En: Déjalo así.
28 N: Leave it like this.

[The nurse then looks down between Guadalupe's legs.]

En: Como la lastimaron, pobrecita. Para acá se la hubieron traído, pobrecita, como la lastiman.
29 N: How they hurt you, poor thing. They should have brought you
30 here, how they hurt you.

[The nurse looks at Guadalupe's family.]

En: Ella se va a quedar hospitalizada oye.
31 N: She is going to be admitted to the hospital, do you hear?

[The nurse leaves to get an IV, and when the phone rings she remains out of the room attending to the call. In the meantime the doctor arrives at 12:31 PM.]

Doctor: Bueno. Vamos a esperar afuerita por favor.
32 Doctor: Okay. Let's wait outside please.

Es: Bueno. Que. Ya la va a atender?
33 H: Okay. What. Are you going to treat her now?

D: Si. Allá afuera esperas un rato.
34 D: Yes. Please wait over there outside for a while.

[The nurse returns.]

En: Ya déjela. ... Si necesitamos algo, allí lo vamos a llamar.
35 N: Go ahead and leave her. ... If we need anything, we will go over
36 there and call you.

Es: Bueno esta bien.
37 H: Okay.

D: Vamos a ver está el cordón allí.
38 D: Let's see if the cord is there.

En: Si … Ah estaba muy pálida antes de dar a luz.
39 N: Yes … Ah, she was really pale before giving birth.

D: Si pero ahorita ya agarró.
40 D: Yes, but only recently did it really get her.

En: Mire como esta de lastimada pobrecita.
41 N: Look at how she is hurt, poor thing.

D: Si por eso le digo que conmigo … va a ser mejor.
42 D: Yep, that's why I say that as far as I'm concerned … it is going
43 to be better—

En: Me cierra la mano.
44 N: Close your hand for me. [The nurse takes a blood draw.]

D: —dejarlas hospitalizadas. Donde vivís?
45 D: —to admit this woman to the hospital. Where do you live?

Guadalupe: En Chupöl.
46 Guadalupe: In Chupöl.

D: Chupöl. Ahora vamos a hacer su ingreso.
47 D: Chupöl. Now we are going to process your admittance.

G: Mhhhh.
48 G: Mmmhhh.

At 12:32 PM the doctor and the nurse leave. She goes to get an IV and
he goes to get his paper work. He stops and talks to her family, who is
waiting outside of the examination area.

D: Ya se va a quedar, oyó?
49 D: She is going to stay, did you hear?

[When he gets no response from the family, he repeats himself.]

D: Se va a quedar hospitalizada hoy.
50 D: She is going to have to be admitted today.

Es: Y por lo menos cuando voy a traer?
51 H: And at the very least when will I come and get her?

D: Mira, mañana que pasan a ver los doctores ***, y si todo esta bien
mañana le dan salida.
52 D: Look, tomorrow the doctors are going to stop by and see her
53 [words unclear], and if everything is okay tomorrow, they will
54 discharge her.

[The nurse returns and administers the IV while the doctor continues talking to the family.]

En: No se vaya a mover.
55 N: Don't move.

G: Vaya.
56 G: Okay.

En: Pinchoncito.
57 N: A little pinch.

[Meanwhile the doctor is walking through the room with his papers, talking to her family.]

D: Hay que dejarle medicina para que no se le vaya a infectar allí.
58 D: You have to administer medicine so that she doesn't get infected
59 there.

[The doctor re-enters the space with Guadalupe and begins the admission paperwork.]

D: Como se llama?
60 D: What's your name?

[Guadalupe supplies her full name again.]

D: Chupöl. ... Chichi?
61 D: Chupöl. ... Chichi?

D: Cuántos años Guadalupe?
62 D: How old, Guadalupe?

G: Tiene 18.
63 G: She is 18 [sic].

D: Sabe leer y escribir?
64 D: Do you know how to read and write?

G: Si.
65 G: Yes.

D: A que grado llegaste?
66 D: What grade did you get to?

G: Cuarto.
67 G: Fourth.

D: Cuarto primera?
68 D: Fourth grade of elementary?

G: Si.
69 G: Yes.

D: Estas casada o unida?
70 D: Are you married or in a civil union?

G: Casada.
71 G: Married.

[The doctor starts to put on his latex gloves.]

D: Aborto no has tenido?
72 D: Have you ever had a miscarriage?

G: Que?
73 G: What?

D: Aborto. Que se te han venido muchachitos antes. No?
74 D: Miscarriage. Have you ever received children in your belly be-
75 fore. No?

G: No.
76 G: No.

[With his gloves on, the doctor begins his exam.]

En: Es el primer niño eso.
77 N: This is your first child.

D: Es el primero.
78 D: This is your first.

G: Si.
79 G: Yes.

D: Y esta vivo el bebé?
80 D: And is the baby alive?

G: Si.
81 G: Yes.

D: Si. Todo normal con el niño?
82 D: Yes. Everything normal with the baby?

G: Si.
83 G: Yes.

D: Tiene la presión Ana [referring to the nurse]?
84 D: Do you have the blood pressure, Ana?

E: Si, 170.
85 E: Yes, 170.

D: A que hora nació el niño?
86 D: What time was the baby born?

G: Hmmm?
87 G: Hmmmm?

D: A que hora nace el niño?
88 D: What time is the baby born?

G: Que hora?
89 G: What time?

D: Si.
90 D: Yes.

G: A las diez y media.
91 G: At 10:30.

D: Diez y media.
92 D: 10:30.

[The doctor finishes his exam and disposes of the gloves, and the nurse asks him about the dose of medicine.]

En: [A Doctor] Cuanto entonces? Diez y 75 o cinco 75?
93 N: [To the doctor] How much, then? Ten and seventy-five or five
94 and seventy-five?

D: Hagamos con 5.
95 D: Let's do it with five.

En: A bueno
96 N: Oh, Okay.

[At 12:36 PM the nurse shoots a narcotic into Guadalupe's IV. The doctor and the nurse leave. Guadalupe's husband and mother-in-law are waiting outside of the curtain. After just a little while Guadalupe starts to grunt and mumble in a slurred voice. Immediately, her husband goes through the curtain to try to talk to her. She is very drugged and not able to respond to him. The husband, who does not know that she has been given a large dose of Demerol, immediately goes to find the doctor. He attempts to engage the doctor, who does not pay attention to him, but rather calls the nurse. Three minutes have passed since they left Guadalupe.]

D: Vamos Ana!
97 D: Come on, Ana!

En: Voy.
98 E: I'm coming.

D: Vamos a ver como esta ahorita.
99 D: Let's see how you are [or how she is] now.

[Guadalupe groans and mumbles. The nurse arrives. The doctor begins a manual extraction of the placenta.]

En: Ya ahorita va a estar.
100 N: In a minute it will be all over.

[At 12:42 PM the doctor pulls the placenta out of Guadalupe.]

En: Ya está. Ya estuvo, ya estuvo.
101 N: It's out. That was it, that was it.

[Guadalupe groans. The doctor is examining the placenta.]

En: Ya estuvo.
102 N: That was it.

D: Bueno. Ya está completa entonces. No hay lesión aquí. De membranas enteras. Placenta está completa.
103 D: Good. Then that is done. There are no lesions here. The mem-
104 branes are whole. The placenta is complete.

[At 12:43 PM the doctor leaves and goes to wash his hands. The nurse cleans Guadalupe up, and then covers her with a sheet and leaves to get an injectable antibiotic. At 12:45 the nurse returns to administer the injection, at which point Guadalupe's husband stops her and asks about his wife.]

Es: Enh, disculpe, pongamos cuanto, cuanto se se va a quedarnos?
105 H: Ahh, excuse me, let's speculate how much, how much is she,
106 are we staying?[6]

En: Si, se queda.
107 N: Yes, she stays.

Es: Lo que pasa es que esta el bebe en la casa.
108 H: What's going on is that the baby is at home.

En: Pues tráiganse el bebe en la tarde.
109 N: Well, bring the baby in the afternoon.

Es: Lo que pasa nosotros venimos directos, usted ya no, ya no, ahora …
110 N: What's going on we came directly, you are not going to, going
111 to, now …

En: Y entonces que quiere usted?
112 N: And so what do you want?

Es: Tal vez, o sea, pongamos, aunque tarde ...
113 H: Maybe, I mean, let's say, even if it were late ...

En: Como?
114 N: What?

Es: Aun que tarde, pero nos vamos como el bebe esta en la casa. O sea, aunque tarde.
115 H: Even if it were late, but we leave since the baby is left at home.
116 I mean, even if it is late.

En: Ay. Entonces hable con el doctor porque ella se tiene que quedar porque esta muy lastimada de aquí de su parte, pero si ustedes se la quieren llevar tiene que firmar un libro y se la pueden llevar pero eso es peligroso porque se le puede infectar.
117 N: Ahh. Then you should speak with the doctor because she
118 needs to stay because she is very hurt down there in her private
119 parts, but if you all want to take her you have to sign the book
120 and you can take her but that is dangerous because it could get
121 infected.

Es: A ya. De todo modo por eso. Entonces. Pongamos cuanto, cuanto tiempo va a tardar?
122 H: Uh huh. In any case, because of that. So. Let's say how much,
123 how much time is it going to take?

En: Si todo esta bien, posiblemente mañana se la den. Esta muy pálida a ver si no esta con anemia.
124 N: If everything is okay, they will possibly let her go tomorrow.
125 She is very pale let's see if she doesn't have anemia.

[At this point the doctor calls the nurse from the other room and she turns and leaves. When she goes Guadalupe's husband lets out a deep breath. He then goes and talks to his parents. The nurse returns to Guadalupe's bed.]

En: Hágase para acá. Espere, espéreme un ratito.
126 N: Scoot over here. Wait, wait for me for a second.

[At 12:48 PM the nurse emerges from behind the curtain and calls for Guadalupe's family.]

En: Viene a ayudarme. Entonces que van a hacer? La va a dejar?
127 N: Come and help me. So what are you going to do? Are you go-
128 ing to leave her?

Es: Si. Creo que si. La vamos a dejar.
129 H: Yes. I think so. We are going to leave her.

En: Es para el bienestar de ella y para el bienestar de ustedes. Oye?
130 N: It's for her own good and your good also. Do you hear?

Es: Si. Eso es ... es lo que pensamos.
131 H: Yes. It is ... it is what we think.

En: Va. Ayúdame. Pues, la vamos a pasar para acá.
132 N: Okay. Help me. Well, we are going to move her over here
133 [onto the stretcher].

Es: Vaya. Aquí la voy a agarrar. ... Ya.
134 H: Okay. I'm going to grab her here. ... Ready.

En: No. haga de aquí, ve? De aquí, de la cintura porque sino no la
vamos a poder.
135 N: No. Do it from here, see? From here, at her waist because if
136 not we won't be able to do it.

Es: Aquí o sea, la misma?
137 H: Here, I mean, the same?

En: Si si. Porque todo resulta muy manchada.
138 N: Yes, yes. Because everything will wind up really stained.

Es: ha. ... Todo modos.
139 H: Oh. ... Anyhow.

En: Saque, saque todo eso.
140 N: Take away, take away all of that.

Es: Todo modo no va a necesitar todito porque tenemos la ropa así.
141 H: In any case, she won't need everything because we have her
142 clothes like this.

En: No. No, porque ahorita se queda con la ropa de aquí.
143 N: No. No, because now she has to remain with the clothes from
144 here.

Es: Aquí, aquí se queda. No, aquí?
145 H: Here, here she remains. No, here?

En: No. Ahorita me la voy a llevar para adentro.
146 N: No. Soon I will take her inside [to the ward].

[The nurse leaves and attends to other matters. Guadalupe's husband
stays with his wife. At 12:55 PM Guadalupe's husband goes back to
find the nurse.]

Es: Disculpe yo, yo podía dejarme con ella?
147 H: Excuse me and I, I could stay with her?

En: No. No se puede ...
148 N: No. No one can ...

Es: No se puede.
149 H: No one can.

En: ... hay una comadrona allí que les ayuda. Oye, no tengan pena.
150 N: ... there is a midwife there that helps them. Listen, don't
151 worry.

Es: No, lo que pasa que nosotros estábamos pensando ahorita, talvez
podía mandar a una mi hermana, allí si?
152 H: No, what's going on is that we were just thinking that maybe
153 I could send one of my sisters, in that way, yes?

En: No. Ahorita ya no se esta permitiendo, porque ya hay una comadrona que habla dialecto, que las ayuda que ... todo, no hay necesidad que se quede ninguno. A las 4:00 de la tarde cuando venga el
medico de turno, ustedes le hablan y el dice que sí, entonces sí, pero
de lo contrario, no se está dejando a ninguno.
154 N: No. Right now no one is being permitted to, because there is
155 already a midwife who speaks dialect, that helps the women, that
156 ... everything, there is no reason for anyone to stay. At 4:00 PM
157 when the doctor on call comes in, you all can talk to him, and if he
158 says yes, then yes, but to the contrary, no one is allowed to stay.

Es: O sea, mañana?
159 H: I mean, tomorrow?

En: Hoy en la tarde.
160 N: This afternoon.

Es: Hoy en la tarde va a salir?
161 H: This afternoon she's going to go?

En: Nooooo.
162 N: Nooooo.

Es: Como así?
163 H: How is that?

En: Miré pues, no se esta dejando a ninguna persona que se queden
aquí con las pacientes porque hay una ... hay una comadrona que
habla en dialecto, que las ayuda... que si necesita alguien que habla
en dialecto, entonces ella las ayuda.

164 N: Look here, no one is permitted to stay here with the patients
165 because there is a midwife who speaks in dialect, who helps them
166 ... if one needs someone who speaks in dialect, then she helps
167 them.

Es: Ahhh.
168 H: Ohh.

En: Entonces a las 4:00 de la tarde si ustedes vienen a hablar con el
medico, si el dice que si, entonces si, si no, de lo contrario, no hay
necesidad.
169 N: Then at 4:00 PM if you all come and speak to the doctor, if he
170 says yes, then yes, if not, to the contrary, it is not necessary.

[The nurse turns and talks to another worker. At 1:10 PM she returns
and they all leave with the nurse wheeling Guadalupe to the maternity ward.]

Understanding the Interaction

I want to start the analysis of the conversation by pointing to two
larger issues that frame it: the use of Spanish language, and the issue of transport. The nurse asserts her position of authority almost
from the start. In Spanish when you speak to another person, you
can "treat" them familiarly or formally. While the nurse uniformly
uses formal address to converse with the doctor, she does not with
the family. Indeed, she often mixes formal (*usted*) and informal (*tú*)
address when talking to Guadalupe and her family, even in the same
sentence. Guadalupe's husband, the only one to address the nurse,
always addresses her formally.

It becomes more and more obvious as the conversation unfolds
that Guadalupe and her family have little dominion over Spanish.
Neither her mother-in-law nor her father-in-law ever utter a word
of Spanish the entire time that they are in the ER. Despite her four
years of primary school Guadalupe herself has a difficult time with
Spanish. When the doctor asks her how old she is (line 62) she re-
plies in third person singular rather than first person (line 63). She
has a difficult time understanding his questions. In lines 72–76 the
doctor asks her about past miscarriages, a question she does not understand. In lines 86–91, where the doctor questions her about the
time at which the baby was born, she again has a difficult time understanding. The doctor switches from past tense to present tense,
hoping to simplify the question for her. Most everything else that

she says is "yes." In addition, Guadalupe's husband translates all of the nurse's requests for her.

Her husband, who has the most command of Spanish, nonetheless reveals several times that his linguistic skills are also poor. When the nurse first asks how many babies Guadalupe has (lines 1–5), her husband mixes up the gendered articles. The nurse first uses *niños* (children), which is masculine, and Guadalupe's husband answers the question with a feminine adjective. The nurse then repeats the exact same question but uses *bebé* (baby) another masculine noun, to make sure that he is answering her question and not some other. Despite modeling again the correct masculine article, Guadalupe's husband still responds with a feminine adjective. His lack of ability to negotiate the situation well is also evident when he attempts to ask the nurse how long Guadalupe needs to stay, and if they can go home that day (lines 105–121). In line 105 he asks either an explicitly vague or just incomprehensible question, which the nurse chooses to interpret as an inquiry into whether or not Guadalupe must stay, ignoring the two times he said "how long" in the utterance. Again, when they are all changing Guadalupe's clothes (lines 141–145) the conversation is strained. In line 143 the nurse uses the verb *quedarse* (which most literally means "to remain"), to refer to the fact that Guadalupe has to remain in the hospital clothes and has no need for her family to leave her own clothes. Guadalupe's husband repeats two words—*aquí* [here] and *quedarse*—from the nurse's utterances, directly after she finishes. However, he recovered a different meaning of the verb altogether. Now, instead of referring to keeping the clothes "from here," he is referring to his wife staying here. The nurse then tells him that his wife will go to the ward (not remain in the ER). Finally, in the end of the conversation (lines 147–162), when Guadalupe's husbands wants to know if they can have someone stay with her, the conversation again becomes strained. The nurse explains to Guadalupe's husband that when the doctor-on-call arrives at 4:00 PM, they can ask his permission to stay. After finishing her instructions, Guadalupe's husband asks for a clarification of the time, and then when the nurse repeats that it is today in the afternoon, Guadalupe's husband, immediately interprets this as meaning that Guadalupe will be released today in the afternoon. The nurse becomes frustrated and says a very long "nooooo," and explains the entire process over again.

The importance of Guadalupe's family's lack of facility for speaking Spanish does not lie in the miscommunication that results, but rather in the power differential that it both creates and indexes. Despite the fact that it is obvious from the first utterances that there might be some language difficulties, the nurse never acknowledges the issue. Indeed, there are no translators at the hospital; the nurse is a monolingual Spanish speaker and nearly every patient that she sees has some problem with Spanish. As an individual there is nothing that she can do about that. But the fact that it is assumed that Spanish is the language of conversation in the hospital, and at no time does anyone attempt to address the nurse in K'iche', nor assume that someone should be there to help them in their own language are really the important points here.

Bourdieu (1991) helps us understand why this might be through his idea of symbolic capital. While it is quite obvious that in Guatemala, there is a connection between resource distribution and native language of the speaker (i.e., Spanish speakers control most resources), this is not because Spanish speakers are more adept communicators. Rather than theorizing language as a transparent mode of communication, Bourdieu recognizes that language itself is a resource or good. An individual can use language, his/her symbolic capital, in order to gain access to more tangible goods. Linguistic practices will vary throughout society and access to certain practices will be stratified. Which variety of linguistic practices are privileged depends on which are legitimated by institutions of the State. These linguistic practices hold no power by themselves, but rather only reflect the influence of the groups that use them. Nevertheless, these prestige forms are promoted by institutions (like schools) as inherently better or more correct practice. Rather than question its legitimacy, people without access to symbolic capital esteem it.

Using Bourdieu as a guide helps us appreciate the myriad disadvantages that not being a Spanish speaker produces. At the level of signs, Guadalupe's family's lack of Spanish skills signals their position in society. Despite the fact that Spanish is the esteemed linguistic practice, and that this practice is legitimized and reinforced by the Guatemalan educational system, the press, the government, etc., neither Guadalupe nor her family have had enough access to it to master it. Their exclusion from this prestige dialect, then, indexes their overall limited access to most resources. In sum, Spanish and K'iche' are not equal. K'iche' speakers should be able to carry on in Spanish if they want service. For this reason, at no time does the nurse slow down, or even acknowledge in an empathetic way that Guadalupe or her husband might be having difficulty speaking or understanding Spanish. Instead, she simply expects them to be able to. And when Guadalupe's husband really fails to understand the direct message of how things work in the hospital, it elicits a frustrated "Noooooooo" from the nurse.

Another issue that remains unarticulated but is actually central to Guadalupe's story is that of transport. To get from Chichicastenango to the Sololá hospital on public transport involves taking a bus from Chichi to Los Encuentros (about an hour), changing buses, and then traveling from Los Encuentros to Sololá (usually a ten- to thirty-minute wait and then another hour of transit time), and then frequently changing to another bus to get to the hospital (another possible 30 minutes of wait and 5 minutes of transit time). I have not been to Chupöl, but getting from Chupöl to Chichi would involve *at least* another bus ride. In addition to the number of connections they would have to make, Guatemalan buses are notoriously packed. Transport is provided in old Blue Bird school buses, where three adults must share one seat. Then extra passengers are crammed into the aisle. They are tighter than a subway car at rush hour. In short, it would have been nearly impossible for them to have brought Guadalupe to the hospital with public transport. But to rent a private vehicle is a luxury and costs at least several days pay.[7]

The problems with transport provide a backdrop for the interaction. In addition to the fact that Guadalupe's family does not want to leave her alone (as demonstrated by the offer to find a female relative to stay with her), they also have to consider the cost of transporting her. If she does not leave today, then they will have to contract private transport again to pick her up.[8] If she does leave today, it is possible that the longer she stays in the hospital, and the longer the drivers have to remain waiting, the more expensive the trip. Guadalupe's husband inquires a number of times how much time his wife will have to spend in the hospital, but is continually rebuffed. What is important to the nurse is that Guadalupe needs to be admitted and will be released when she is better. But her husband needs an answer to this question to be able to make the best investment of his resources (i.e., perhaps tell her uncle to go ahead and return quickly).

Another transport-related issue concerns the baby: Guadalupe gave birth that morning, yet the baby is at home with her mother. Guadalupe's husband tells the nurse twice that they would like to take her home, even if it were late that night, because the baby is at home without her. The nurse, who does not doubt the logic of the fact that the baby and mother should be together, tells her husband to bring the baby to her during visiting hours that evening. While well-meaning, this suggestion is also impractical. For the same rea-

sons that it would be difficult to bring Guadalupe to the hospital on
public transport, it would be difficult with the baby. The conditions
of the buses are hard and less than day–old newborns might not be
up to them. It is doubtful that any good parent would allow such
a young baby out of the house. Infant mortality in these areas is
high. New mothers room in with their babies for seven days doing
absolutely nothing. There is no passing around of the baby, and no
constant entourage of visitors. Babies that young are far more vulnerable to sickness, and, people believe, to evil eye. Accordingly, it
would be a terrible idea to bring a newborn on a packed bus, since
the attention that it would draw could easily result in some passenger unintentionally passing it the evil eye. And, there are the prac-
ticalities of time. Buses do not serve rural communities round the
clock. Rather they tend to leave them in the morning and return in
the afternoon. It is, therefore, not a given that even if Guadalupe's
husband called their village and was able to communicate the message to bring the baby, a bus would be available to bring them to
the hospital. So bringing the baby would probably involve renting
another private vehicle, a prohibitive expense.

In sum, the nurse never seems to acknowledge that transportation issues might form real constraints for Guadalupe's family. Her
family, obviously, never directly brings it up either, but rather inti-
mates. For example, in line 110 Guadalupe's husband tells the nurse
that they arrived "directly," that is to say, with a private car. By not
recognizing that transport and the expense of transport is a difficult
issue for them at these points, the nurse eliminates any comfortable
space where this issue could be brought up. Indeed when she says
"they should have brought you earlier," she again negates the issue
of transport as being a limitation that must be negotiated. In this
way she asserts that transport shouldn't be an issue, and she effec-
tively neutralizes any of the family's practical arguments as to why
Guadalupe should go home today.

In this interaction Guadalupe's family indexes their own social
position over and over again. They cannot speak Spanish. They cannot afford much private transport. Yet, by not acknowledging these
facts publicly, and in fact intimating that neither should be an issue, the nurse implicitly negates their appropriateness. As a result,
the factor that most heavily weighs on Guadalupe's situation, that
is her family's lack of access to capital, symbolic or otherwise, is ignored, and her situation must be negotiated without recognizing
these limitations as legitimate constraints. In short, even it if is okay
to be poor and indigenous, it's not okay to *act* poor (e.g., not pay

for several private trips to the hospital) or indigenous (e.g., speak K'iche').

I now want to go back to the interaction and look at specific utterances both to better illustrate how the nurse molds the conversations to very clearly reflect her judgments of Guadalupe's treatment thus far, and how she tries to ensure that Guadalupe remain in the hospital. The first line of communication that can be heard when everyone enters the ER is the nurse asking for the number of children Guadalupe has had. But how many children she has is really not relevant to her retained placenta.[9] Only then does the nurse actually look at Guadalupe and cry out:

En: ¡Huy! Esta superpalida usted. ... Ha sangrado mucho? Ha sangrado mucho?
8 N: Oooh! You are incredibly pale. ... Did you bleed a lot? Did she
9 bleed a lot?

Again, it is difficult to read this as a neutral question. The implication is that if Guadalupe did bleed a lot, then her family did not take good care of her. Therefore, her husband answers that she did not, to which the nurse rejoins:

En: O estaba muy pálida cuando estaba embarazada?
11 N: Or was she really pale when she was pregnant?

If Guadalupe did not bleed a lot during the birth, then the nurse assumes that she must have had this condition the entire time that she was pregnant. The nurse insinuates that Guadalupe's health is in a generally poor state and her family was unable to take good care of her. With this line, the nurse enters into fact that Guadalupe was too pale. Guadalupe's husband does not deny that she was pale, rather he attempts to agree with the nurse, but lessen the severity of the problem.

Es: Si estaba un poquito pálida.
12 H: Yes, she was a little pale.

But when the nurse and the doctor were treating Guadalupe, the nurse reports that Guadalupe was *very* pale before giving birth (line 39).

If it was not already obvious that the nurse saw Guadalupe's homebirth as harmful, it becomes emphatically clear as she is helping to change Guadalupe's clothes. She positions herself at Guadalupe's feet, and then looks between her legs. When she does, she exclaims:

En: Como la lastimaron, pobrecita. Para acá se la hubieron traído, pobrecita, como la lastiman.
26 N: How they hurt you, poor thing. They should have brought you
here, how they hurt you.[10]

Who exactly "they" are in this statement is unclear. It could be the
midwives, Guadalupe's family, or a combination of both. Regardless,
the important point is that the nurse is asserting again that Guadalupe has been abused. Her condition is not the result of her pregnancy or birth, but rather the result of the injury that she suffered
at her family's or midwife's hands. When she says, finally, "*como la
lastiman*" in present tense, she indicates that the injury is continuing
or widespread, but not confined only to Guadalupe's past.

The theme of Guadalupe's injury continues throughout the interaction. Later (lines 113–116), when her family is asking when she
will be released, the nurse tells them to talk with the doctor "*porque
ella se tiene que quedar porque esta muy lastimada de aquí de su parte*"
(because she is very hurt down there in her private parts). After
Guadalupe is admitted to the maternity ward I asked her family if
they understood why the doctor said that Guadalupe needed to stay
in the hospital. Her husband responded that she needed to stay because "*le hizo algo malo y lastimó la parte* [sic]" (she[11] did something
wrong and hurt her private parts). I then asked them to explain to
me what treatment she had received from the doctor so far. He told
me that they had been unable to talk to Guadalupe,[12] so they didn't
know if the doctor extracted the placenta or how it went.

In the end, Guadalupe's hurt "privates" become the focus of her
need for medical care. The nurse's position was that because Guadalupe had been hurt, she had to be left in the hospital. In reality
it is difficult to understand how Guadalupe had been hurt. In general, midwives do not attempt to perform manual extraction, nor
to remove the placenta by force. Many midwives told me that the
placenta can migrate upward through the woman, and the force of
pulling the cord could be similar to stretching a rubber band: if you
stretch the cord and then let go, the placenta will shoot back up
into the trunk of a woman. If Guadalupe had been bruised or swollen by repeated attempts to extract the placenta, someone would
have asked who it was that was trying to extract it.[13] This question
never came up. When the doctor finished with the extraction of
the placenta he reported that there were no lesions or tears to be
repaired in her vagina (line 103). The doctor himself said that Guadalupe needed to be admitted to prevent an infection from taking

hold (lines 58–59), not because she was hurt. The nurse also knew that infection was the issue (lines 120–121).

Guadalupe's family obviously came to the hospital seeking help to remove the placenta, and it was their desire that they be able to take Guadalupe home that day, even if it meant waiting until the night. Their ability to secure their wishes was obscured by their lack of facility with Spanish, as discussed above, but also by the fact that the treatment that Guadalupe was receiving was never discussed with them. They were, therefore, never given an opportunity to agree or disagree. Instead, the treatment options were presented to them as letting her get treated, i.e., leaving her there, or not letting her get treated, i.e., taking her home that night. As the specifics of her treatment were never broached (i.e., we will have to give her a sedative and manually extract the placenta), the implication was that the staff knew what was best for her, and the family had nothing to contribute to the discussion. Indeed, this view point was shored up in line 130 where the nurse responded to the news that they were going to leave Guadalupe:

En: Es para el bienestar de ella y para el bienestar de ustedes. Oye?
130 N: It's for her own good and your good also. Do you hear?

"Skilled" Attendance

In this chapter I have presented a detailed account of an interaction between a K'iche' family seeking emergency obstetric care, and the health workers whom they encounter in the hospital. Discourse analysis is an excellent tool to expose the subtle mechanisms that interlocutors employ in their struggle to achieve their agendas. It also can be used to show how many of the important mechanisms and events are beyond the conscious control of the participants, but are instead habitually ingrained modes of interaction. Rather than painting a picture of the hospital as a bad place where poorly intentioned people work, I have tried to use discourse analysis to show how the interactions are mutually produced (not just dictated by the healthcare workers), and the ways in which clients collude (as well as resist) in their own subjugation. The interaction detailed above also has helped to demonstrate why going to the hospital is frequently thought of as the last option for poor indigenous people, and why the points that are uncomfortable in the delivery of care are so difficult to change.

Reviewing an interaction at such close detail also gives us important information about how the central message of the global campaign to promote Safe Motherhood—that we need "skilled attendance"—can be deployed by health workers. Privileging skilled attendance obviously fits well into the Guatemalan landscape. In this example, the idea of skilled attendance is used to denigrate the homecare that women receive in their villages. Indeed, the message seems to be so appealing to this health worker that instead of predicating her message about Guadalupe's need to stay in the hospital on the more legitimate biomedical explanation, she instead invokes the discourse of skilled attendance.

This example has given us some insight into the unintended, but perhaps not so unanticipated (Kruske and Barclay 2004), consequences of global efforts to make pregnancy safer. Messages and policies certainly do enter receptive and even welcome fields, but these fields are inevitably characterized by their own conflicts and tensions. Yet the assumptions embodied by the idea of "skilled attendance" do not stray far from decades of imagining women who do the jobs of iyom (Pinto 2008), or imagining how to improve attendance (Justice 1986; Pigg 1997). What we have lacked has been any critical, empirical examination of what the emphasis on "skilled attendance" has meant to women and their families on the ground.

Chapter 3

GLOBAL SAFE MOTHERHOOD AND MAKING LOCAL PREGNANCY SAFER

THE SPIN AND WHAT IT COVERS UP

I was quite taken aback the day that I typed "safemotherhood.org" into my web browser, hit Enter, and the page was no longer there. Thinking that I had typed the name incorrectly, I tried again. I was only convinced that it was really gone after I searched for the address on Google, got the non-existent page, but was able to see what I was looking for in the cached page. Could the Safe Motherhood Initiative just disappear? What is the point of erasing the page? Why was it later recreated, but without any useful links to past pages or to the new initiatives that had absorbed it?

In researching efforts to decrease maternal mortality, I have found that the official materials (web pages, reports, and documents put out by international organizations and NGOs) have done little to help me understand the problems and complications that make decreasing maternal mortality so difficult. Instead, the official accounts of Safe Motherhood are predicated on a particular static timeline that starts in 1987 when the Safe Motherhood Initiative was born. With every event and year that ensues we are led to believe that we are moving closer and closer to the final endpoint: significantly reducing maternal mortality.

The timeline depiction hasn't helped my understanding because it is a heavily biased portrayal of events, or, in simpler language, it is spin. I start this chapter by laying out some of the most basic information about international attempts to make pregnancy and birth safer around the world, both to orient the reader, and to explore what the spin (the timeline) looks like. It is actually quite easy to see that a large amount of important information has been extruded from the story of safe motherhood[1] in order to make the timeline. But I show here that we can only understand how and why safe motherhood has been spun the way it has by paying attention to for whom the spin is being spun.

The central tension facing practitioners and policy makers in many arenas of global health is how to maintain safe motherhood among the important global health initiatives that investors (primarily governments and donors) prioritize as "making a difference." Potential donors determine just how good of an investment it is by both the general trends in global health, and by what alternative initiatives and programs might be available to fund. For example, one of the major problems that safe motherhood must contend with is that of numbers—how many women actually die? It is incredibly difficult to get accurate counts of who dies a pregnancy-related death because death certificates frequently underreport maternal death, regardless of whether they are filled out by bureaucrats or medical practitioners (Deneux-Tharaux et al. 2005). Programs aimed at curbing infant mortality do not face the same burdens, as all lifeless infant bodies count, and consequently, it is easier to make a solid case for the dire scope of the problem. It is also more difficult for safe motherhood programs to show an effect since they lack an accurate measure of maternal mortality in the first place (Fauveau and Donnay 2006). The spin, then, must work to favorably position efforts to decrease maternal mortality vis-à-vis other global health initiatives, because in actuality, whether or not investors are willing to give more than token money to try to make pregnancy safer is uncertain.

While the intentional effect of the spin is to generate additional funding, I argue in this chapter that the spin has played a significant role in making safe motherhood a doomed initiative. Because the spin generates funding, it also generates funding priorities. In the second part of the chapter I look at how policy initiatives fomented through the global spin hit the ground in Guatemala. More specifically, I explore the role of midwives in Sololá to show how the translation of the spin into program priorities has arguably endangered the departmental effort to decrease maternal mortality. Finally, I look at how the Safe Motherhood campaign plays out in the village. Despite the fact that Safe Motherhood was probably one of the top-funded programs in Sololá, in the villages where I interviewed I found that women were completely unaware of and unsympathetic to the campaign. I argue that the heavily top-down structure of Safe Motherhood, which the spin necessitates, actually serves as a barrier to the legitimacy of global efforts to decrease maternal mortality.

From the Safe Motherhood Initiative to Making Pregnancy Safer: A Sketch of the Timeline[2]

Oddly enough, there was no united, international effort to address the problem of maternal mortality until the 1980s. Carla AbouZahr (2003), who worked for the WHO on Safe Motherhood for almost two decades, points to two major factors that galvanized a global movement to deal with maternal mortality. International organizations didn't even know the scope of the problem of maternal mortality until changes in statistical methods during the 1980s made possible a somewhat more accurate accounting of pregnancy-related death. The first international estimates were completed in the middle of that decade. At the same time, Allan Rosenfield and Deborah Maine (1985), two researchers from Columbia University, pushed to theoretically redefine maternal health as a field in its own right. They argued that while on paper maternal and child health (MCH) were international priorities, in reality maternal health was only addressed as a factor that could enable children's health.

The Safe Motherhood Initiative (SMI) was the product of the international community's first attempts to delineate a maternal health agenda. In 1987, three UN agencies interested in maternal health sponsored what is referred to as the Nairobi Conference. Together with two other important international organizations, Planned Parenthood International and the Population Council, they outlined a broad agenda for how to decrease global maternal mortality by 50 percent by the year 2000. This agenda, which became known as the SMI, outlined fourteen broad measures to reduce maternal mortality, such as improving family planning services, women's education, primary healthcare, and women's general status in society. The attendants at the conference officially became known as the Safe Motherhood Inter-Agency Group (IAG).

Despite this great stride toward finally paying attention to mothers' health, the first decade of the SMI brought little progress in terms of lowering rates of maternal mortality. Maine and Rosenfield (1999) argued that this failure of the SMI stemmed from a lack of clarity in its agenda. Any government that had a program to improve some aspect of women's lives could claim to be implementing the SMI without doing anything different. Ann M. Starrs (2006) points out that the priorities for the first decade of the SMI were actually determined by "the global commitment to primary health-care."[3] Following this commitment, community-based interventions that attempted to improve prenatal care, or those that worked with traditional midwives[4] (Kwast 1993) were the most widely implemented strategies to decrease maternal mortality.

Why did these strategies lead to naught? The first major argument made was that while prenatal care is valuable, it is not a particularly useful tool for preventing maternal mortality (Rohde 1995). Practitioners cannot reliably predict birthing problems through prenatal contact with pregnant women. Using the example of a cohort of women who experienced obstructed birth, Alicia Ely Yamin and Deborah Maine (1999) illustrate how risk profiling during the prenatal period is not effective. They cite a study of 3,614 pregnant women in Zaire who received prenatal risk screening during their care visits. The researchers found that women with previous birthing problems were nine times more likely to experience an obstructed birth as women with no history of previous problems. While this would seem to indicate practitioners could use a history of previous births to successfully identify women at risk for birthing problems, a closer look shows us that they cannot. Although a higher percentage of women with previous problems experienced an obstructed birth, in absolute numbers more than two times as many women who had no prior history of poor outcomes experienced an obstructed birth during the study (see table 1). In sum, risk profiling correctly identifies a small percentage of a small percentage of women who have an increased risk, but it fails to identify the vast majority of women who will experience birthing problems.

The second major argument as to why the SMI did not lower rates of maternal mortality in its first decade is that working with traditional midwives is not effective in reducing maternal mortality.

TABLE 1. History of previous birthing problems as a predictor of actual difficulties. (Kasongo Project Team 1984; as cited in Yamin and Maine 1999:571)

	History of previous birthing problems	No history of previous birthing problems	Total
Obstructed labor this time	15	36	51
Unobstructed labor this time	141	3422	3563
Total	156	3458	3614

Sue Kruske and Lesley Barcaly (2004) outline how the World Health Organization, in particular, championed the training of traditional birth attendants through the 1970s and 80s. Yet, by 1996 traditional birth attendants were classified by the WHO as unskilled attendants, and all efforts shifted to working only with "skilled" attendants (i.e., those who have biomedical credentials, not just workshop training in biomedical obstetrics). Starrs (1998) summarizes a popular argument concerning traditional birth attendants' ability to only reduce post-partum hemorrhage and infection, and inability to address the remaining majority of primary causes of maternal mortality (i.e., eclampsia, obstructed birth, or unsafe abortion that require surgeries, drug regimes, or blood transfusions). Furthermore, though traditional birth attendants learn new techniques, whether or not they change their practice accordingly is debatable (Jokhio, Winter, and Cheng 2005; Smith et al. 2000; Sibley and Sipe 2004).

Not surprisingly, the second decade of the SMI was decidedly focused on improving skilled attendance at birth,[5] and from about 1999 through 2003 the main intervention advocated by the IAG was to strengthen emergency obstetric care in district health services. The concentration on improving skilled attendance only in emergency obstetric care was championed by Maine and Rosenfield (1999), whose influential argument supporting emergency obstetric care as *the* focus for scarce funds hinges on the contention that most causes of maternal mortality are treatable, and a claim that available research supports the primary role of quality obstetric care in determining death rates.

After five years of investing in emergency obstetric care ostensibly failed to bring about any decrease in maternal mortality, however, support for the intervention waned. In the intervening period the idea of "evidence-based" practice had been exported from medicine into public health promotion (Green 2006; Klein 2000). The gold standard for evidence was a randomized control trial design. Not surprisingly, then, Suellen Miller et al. (2003) critiqued the attention to emergency obstetric care as lacking evidence. They viewed the research asserting a relationship between the quality of obstetric care and rates of maternal mortality, which Maine and Rosenfield relied on, as speculative. Indeed, it had been primarily derived from the work of a medical historian who examined the transition in maternal death rates in Britain and the US over one hundred and fifty years, and who argued that the same thing that worked almost one hundred years ago in these countries should work today in developing countries (Loudon 1992, 2000).

The failure of interventions in emergency obstetric care was basically the death knell for the Safe Motherhood Initiative. Policy shifted to bring attention to skilled attendance at birth into bold relief, while emergency obstetric care faded into the background as just one facet of skilled attendance. Nevertheless, the image of the SMI as a program that could really make a difference was tarnished. First, it had convinced funders (and governments) to invest their money in three different interventions (prenatal care, working with midwives, and strengthening emergency obstetric care), none of which singlehandedly decreased maternal mortality. Second, though shifting its emphasis back to skilled attendance at birth did help save face, this policy is not particularly competitive in the funding world.[6] There are, as of yet, no randomized control trials supporting skilled attendance. Evidence-based practice is what funders are seeking, and the SMI was not evidence-based. Wendy Graham (2002:703) describes the problems succinctly: "Skilled attendance at delivery … is now being promoted as a crucial intervention strategy, but again based on plausibility assessment rather than rigorous evaluations showing this to be effective and cost effective in specific settings or health systems. … Without sound evidence for decision making, safe motherhood programme activities … have lacked continuity and engendered uncertainty and disillusionment among governments and donors."

"Uncertainty and disillusionment" with the SMI notwithstanding, by the time that Graham wrote this, the danger of donors completely abandoning the quest to decrease maternal mortality was neither likely nor feasible. In 2000, 189 nations voted to include improving maternal health as the fifth United Nations Millennium Development Goal (MDG), binding the international community to a goal of decreasing maternal mortality by 75 percent by the year 2015. The only indicator cited to monitor progress toward this goal, besides rates of maternal mortality themselves, is increases in rates of skilled attendance (Rosenfield, Maine, and Freedman 2006).[7]

The recapitulation of the SMI's agenda within the MDGs was not, however, enough to save the IAG. The Safe Motherhood website (the most recent version) tells us that in 2004 the Safe Motherhood IAG blended into the Partnership for Safe Motherhood and Newborn Health (no links provided). Searching on Google for the Partnership for Safe Motherhood and Newborn Health, we find out that in 2005 it became one of the constituents of the Partnership for Maternal, Newborn and Child Health (PMNCH), which the WHO backs as the new focal point for making pregnancy safer. The approach of the PMNCH is to recreate the bond between maternal and child health that preceded the SMI, and its goals are programs that offer a continuum of maternal and newborn care (The Partnership for Maternal Newborn and Child Health 2007).

Unraveling the Spin

Why has the history of safe motherhood unfolded the way that it has? The original SMI proposed ten to eighteen different policy platforms to combat maternal mortality. Yet at each step only one or two of these strategies have been pursued. Why have these particular strategies been chosen and not one of the others? And why did the Safe Motherhood website get erased, then reposted, but without any links to the initiative that is replacing it? As I argued in the beginning of this chapter, what has happened in Safe Motherhood has been very much driven by intentions to impress investors. In terms of Safe Motherhood, this means closely aligning the initiative to trends in international health.

Shifts in Safe Motherhood policy have closely mirrored larger shifts in horizontal to vertical and back toward horizontal paradigms of improving health. The "vertical" approach to health development promotes specific disease control programs that frequently are planned at the upper echelons of bureaucracy. The horizontal approach advocates a health sector–wide strategy that uses a "mixed group of disease control/health promoting activities" (Gish 1982).[8] The vertical approach was dominant in international health until the 1970s. The 1978 Alma Ata Conference, sponsored by the same organizations that shaped the SMI, transformed global public health by questioning the focus of international health programs on the curative medical practices that dominated the vertical approach. Instead, at Alma Ata countries overwhelmingly endorsed a focus on factors that more closely influence a population's health, such as clean water or sanitation. Alma Ata also forwarded an agenda of horizontal healthcare that prioritized basic, preventative, primary healthcare over specific disease control initiatives.

While the policy emphasis in the SMI over its first decade was selectively focused, the interventions supported resonated with the "horizontal," comprehensive agenda of Alma Ata. The proceedings from Alma Ata named traditional midwives, who were already present in communities throughout the world, as potential recruits to help in the primary healthcare effort (Kruske and Barclay 2004). Prenatal care was also firmly ensconced within the horizontal agendas of strengthening comprehensive primary healthcare.

Yet, by the end of the first decade of the SMI, the pendulum had swung away from horizontal, and toward vertical approaches in global health writ large. Policy in the SMI, of course, swung with it by introducing an exclusive focus on improving emergency obstetric care. Improving emergency obstetric care is vertical initiative par excellence. It does not strengthen the general provision of health services nor respond to many different diseases or conditions. It is not preventative.[9] Judith Fortenay (2001) articulates well how maternal mortality was positioned to make vertical interventions not only fit, but also appear as a seamlessly logical policy direction: "maternal mortality is perhaps unique among public health problems, in that its reduction depends on the treatment rather than the prevention of illness." I outlined the basic logic behind this argument when I discussed prenatal care above.

Many involved in Safe Motherhood saw clear advantages to selling vertical programmatic approaches to investors.[10] Programmatic approaches provide a concrete point to rally around, provide talking points to create political will (Shiffman 2007; Shiffman and Smith 2007) and distinguish efforts to make pregnancy safer from efforts to reduce infant mortality, for example (Behague and Storeng 2008). In theory it is much easier to measure their effect, since they emphasize technical strategies (such as midwife training or improving infrastructure to respond to obstetric emergencies) and cost-effectiveness.[11]

Yet, the rise of evidence-based public health eroded the ability of Safe Motherhood to realistically promote vertical initiatives. The push for an evidence base more thoroughly concretized the important connection between proven outcomes and getting money from investors. Safe motherhood is at a clear disadvantage, because estimating maternal mortality is notoriously difficult. Much effort has been spent on developing innovative and novel techniques for measurement (Graham 2002; Hill et al. 2007; Graham, Brass, and Snow 1989; Graham et al. 2008), but even in "developed" countries like the United States, records are not that good (Deneux-Tharaux et al. 2005). But without good estimates to begin with, it is impossible to show outcomes.

In Sololá when I first arrived to examine the policy to invest in emergency obstetric care, the comments of one doctor illustrated for me how the lack of reliability threatened the entire SMI. The director of the Ministry of Health had described the extensive documentation to track maternal mortality that was being implemented as part of the program to improve emergency obstetric care.[12] As the doctor pointed out, maternal mortality was bound to go up on paper, since currently there was almost no formal reporting of pregnancy-related death. The success of the policy would be evaluated on outcomes, and, the doctor argued, the numbers would be so skewed that the policy was essentially condemned to failure. What was the logic in this, he asked? Indeed, poor quality of evidence supporting policy initiatives or evaluations of them was a constant problem for the SMI (Miller et al. 2003; Milne et al. 2004; Tita et al. 2007; Abou-Zahr and Wardlaw 2001; Fauveau and Donnay 2006). Yet the SMI itself was eventually discarded, delinked, and erased because of a failure to decrease these ratios.[13]

The recent swing of the pendulum back toward the horizontal approach has potentially allayed many of the problems that the vertically dominated SMI faced. The top-down, vertical approach of the last decade of the SMI is closely allied with neoliberal thought that sees health as a good and prioritizes the cost-effectiveness of producing outcomes. The new strategic initiative of improving the continuum of care for mothers and newborns shifts the focus *from* efficiency and effectiveness back *toward* a commitment to health. In this context, providing good obstetric care becomes an inalienable right[14] not dependent on outcomes.[15]

Abandoning the SMI and pursuing a horizontal, comprehensive approach also potentially heals fragmenting in the field of maternal health. Opposing voices that offered alternative strategies, including those who continually emphasized a comprehensive approach (Campbell and Graham 2006; Donnay 2000; Koblinsky et al. 2006; Tita 2000), detracted from the appeal of the unified, vertical approach that the SMI was selling during its second decade (Bullough et al. 2005; Costello, Azad, and Barnett 2006). While the horizontal approach will not escape critics, it can undoubtedly incorporate diverse perspectives within its practice.

The third decade of our attempts to lower global ratios of maternal mortality is marked by an attempt to erase the past. Those involved in the fight against maternal mortality have shifted their discourse to try to distance maternal health from a "failed" initiative. Rather than saying "safe motherhood," we now read about "safer motherhood" and even more often, "making pregnancy safer." Yet spinning the history of Safe Motherhood in this particular way comes at a price. The spin claims that we know what needs to be done because we have learned from past mistakes. Yet are the mistakes really mistakes? In the next section I look at the cost of the spin around Safe Motherhood that declared working with midwives as a past mistake from which we have moved on.

Safe Motherhood in Guatemala

Until the beginning of the SMI, very little was known about maternal mortality in Guatemala. In the library of San Carlos University, the main university in Guatemala, I found academic theses of thirty-two different medical students who had each pored over registries of a department[16] or a hospital to estimate rates of maternal mortality, but no country-wide survey had ever been attempted. The government itself, using inexact reports from civil registries, estimated that 110–120 women died for every 100,000 births registered. But in 1987 a representative of the Ministry of Health attended the Nairobi Conference, and shortly thereafter, a concerned individual working in the Ministry garnered international funding to undertake the first countrywide survey of maternal mortality (Shiffman and Garcés del Valle 2006). Heraldo Medina-Giron (1989), the doctor who carried out the first survey, settled on a methodology of examining every civil registry from 1988 in every department, and evaluating each death of a woman to see if it was pregnancy-related. He came up with an index of underreporting which ranged from 21.6 percent in the department of Sacatepéquez, to 64.3 percent in Retalhuleu. Calculating the number of deaths per 100,000 births and taking into account the underreporting, he estimated the real rate of maternal mortality in Guatemala was likely to be around 219.

This number that Medina-Giron produced was almost twice what the government had been asserting, but it was difficult for officials to definitively refute the number until the end of the 1990s when USAID funded a second country-wide survey. The report used a different methodology to calculate maternal mortality than did Medina-Giron. First, where Medina-Giron had estimated the number of deaths per 100,000 births, this report estimated the deaths per 100,000 *live* births.[17] Second, where Medina-Giron has used the civil registries (i.e., essentially paper documents), the report got the number of recorded deaths out of a relatively newly implemented computer database system used by the Ministry of Health nationwide. It then used Medina-Giron's estimates of underreporting to adjust the figure. This report calculated ratios of maternal mortality for 1996, 1997, 1998, and estimated that 184, 181, and 186 women died per 100,000 live births respectively (Schieber and Stanton 2000).

But what the Ministry of Health claims as the most thorough nationwide survey of maternal mortality puts the rate of death even lower. This survey, conducted by the Ministry itself with funding from several international NGOs and bilateral agencies (MSPAS

2003), sought to establish the rates of maternal mortality for the year 2000. Like the prior estimate, this survey used statistics from the Ministry of Health computer database system, but it compared those to figures from the Instituto Nacional de Estadística (INE) (National Institute of Statistics) to improve their accuracy. The Ministry then used the same estimates from Medina-Giron to adjust for underreporting. This report found 153 maternal deaths for every 100,000 live births.

What does 110 or 120 or 153 mean? And why is it important? In short, maternal mortality has become a political issue in Guatemala. When the government signed the Peace Accords in 1996 to end a protracted civil war,[18] it promised to reduce rates of pregnancy-related death within the country by 50 percent by the year 2000. While this might seem like a strange item to be detailed in the Peace Accords, creating better, universal healthcare and education was one of the major terms of peace. As the Ministry's most recent report on maternal mortality (MSPAS 2003) showed, not everyone in the nation is at risk. Statistically, a woman who dies a pregnancy-related death in Guatemala is most likely to be an indigenous mother, with little or no education or job, who birthed at home with a traditional midwife. Indeed, the study found that, nationwide, of the 651 pregnancy-related deaths in 2000, only 3 percent of the women had a secondary education or higher. In the introduction to this report the authors outline the important connection between maternal deaths and the State:

> Además de las repercusiones en el seno familiar de la muerte de una madre, la mortalidad maternal es un indicador que refleja el nivel de inequidad y el desarrollo socio económico de los países. Visto desde otro ángulo, la reducción de la mortalidad materna es un indicador sensible del compromiso social con el desarrollo humano. Es por ello que los Acuerdos de Paz lo han incluido como una de las metas sociales del estado.

> In addition to the repercussion on the home front from the death of a mother, maternal mortality is an indicator that reflects the level of inequality and social and economic development of a country. Looked at from another angle, the reduction of maternal mortality is a sensitive indicator of the dedication to human development. It is for this reason that the Peace Accords included it as a social goal of the state (MSPAS 2003, translation by the author).

There is a striking overlap between individuals at risk for a maternal death and those who the government victimized during the

civil war. Thus, within Guatemala, the Ministry of Health is particularly sensitive to the ratio of maternal mortality, as it could be used
as a measure of whether or not the government is living up to its
obligations and, I would argue, how much the State has actually
changed.

So how do we read 153 deaths per 100,000 live births? The first
thing that it says is that rates of maternal mortality are still unaccept-
ably high judged by the standards that the government set for itself
in the 1996 Peace Accords. Due to the Ministry's own 2003 estimates of maternal mortality, the goal of reducing maternal mortality
by half was delayed until 2004. But again, the date came and went
without the goals being achieved. On the other hand, the number
153 relieves pressure, since the Ministry of Health interprets its survey to demonstrate that maternal mortality in Guatemala is fairly
static (read "not getting worse") and claims that the levels found are
commensurate with other countries in similar states of development
(MSPAS 2003).

While the countrywide levels of maternal mortality may be on
par with what is expected for a country like Guatemala, the rates in
Sololá are undoubtedly not. The profile of the "typical" Guatemalan
victim of pregnancy-related death that the Ministry's survey outlined actually fits the vast majority of women birthing in Sololá. Not
surprisingly, then, rates of maternal mortality in Sololá are typically
around three times those estimated for the nation (Schieber and
Stanton 2000; MSPAS 2003; Medina-Giron 1989) and are possibly
up to six times higher than those in the capital, Guatemala City
(World Health Organization et al. 2007).

Because of the desperate situation, Sololá has been the target of
national and international interventions to curb maternal mortality
since 1994. The first full-time program aimed at reducing maternal
mortality was run by a group called MotherCare, which received funding through John Snow Inc. administered through USAID (Mother-
Care et al. 1999). MotherCare was piloted in Guatemala from 1989
through 1994 in Quetzaltenango (MotherCare and USAID 1994).
The grant was then extended for another five years and several more
areas, including Sololá, were added.

MotherCare's strategies for decreasing maternal mortality were
closely aligned with the early SMI. The main focus of the program
centered on midwife training and prenatal care. It worked with biomedical health workers from the Ministry of Health and with the
public in an effort to educate them about maternal mortality. It produced a number of studies (MotherCare et al. 1999; Hurtado 1995)

and educational materials to use in health posts during prenatal counseling visits and also to use in hospitals (MSPAS and Mother-Care 1998; MSPAS, MotherCare, and USAID 1995; MSPAS et al. 1996). As the SMI changed its orientations in the second decade, and prenatal care and working with midwives became mistakes that we learned from, MotherCare eventually lost its contract.

In 1999, Jhpiego, an NGO affiliated with Johns Hopkins, took over the Safe Motherhood campaign in Sololá and it proposed to shift efforts toward improving emergency obstetric care. As a condition of receiving the grant, Jhpiego was asked to employ the MotherCare staff, some of whom had ten years' experience in the area. Jhpiego also worked closely with USAID and the Ministry of Health to execute the program. The intervention to improve emergency obstetric care had a number of facets. The main activities concerned enhancing the district hospital. Both the general practitioners who staffed the emergency room and the nurses attended skill-building sessions where they updated their knowledge about how to respond to an obstetric emergency. The emergency room was outfitted with the most necessary drugs. An additional OB was hired in order to staff the hospital during normal operating hours. Nurses who worked in health centers and health posts were also invited to workshops to improve their skills of responding to and/or diagnosing an obstetric emergency. Another area of major interest for USAID and Jhpiego was to encourage both communities and individuals to prepare better to evacuate emergency obstetric patients. [19] Working through the directorate of the Ministry of Health, the head of each Sololá health district was encouraged to convoke town meetings in each village under their purview to help the town establish an emergency evacuation network. During prenatal care visits women would also receive cards that had the "danger signs" of pregnancy and birth on one side and, on the other, several graphics to help them plan their own emergency evacuations. They were encouraged to save money, find a babysitter for their children, contract transportation, etc., all in advance.

It is in this shift between MotherCare and Jhpiego that we can begin to see how the spin is not just a biased story told about Safe Motherhood, but how that story organizes and directs actions of health workers trying to reduce maternal mortality. As discussed in the previous section, the timeline version of the SMI depicts an "ah-ha" moment at the end of the first decade. Our problem, so the story goes, was that the initiative lacked a defined focus, and we were putting money into things that couldn't have actually reduced

maternal mortality (working with midwives, for example). Investing in emergency obstetric care was presented as a radically different, promising shift in focus. And the money followed this focus.
Donors like John Snow Inc. shifted the terms of their competition
for granting contracts to reflect this new SMI policy. So while there
used to be money in midwives, funding was now only available for
those working to bolster emergency obstetric care.

What this shift meant in practice was that a large part of the work
that Jhpiego staff had to do to promote safe motherhood became
both invisible and unfundable. Jhpiego workers were in no position
to let their relationships with iyoma wane. The iyoma held a vir-
tual monopoly on access to pregnant and birthing women in Sololá,
who vastly preferred the iyoma's services to the biomedical services
available. In Sololá, Ministry of Health department registries show
that over 90 percent of babies are born outside of the hospital; almost all of these births take place with an iyom. In addition, women
who die pregnancy-related deaths are doing so in the village, not in
the hospital.[20] Finally, shift or no shift, there are not enough professional midwives or skilled attendants to deliver all of the pregnant
women.

In short, the success of using emergency obstetric care to decrease
maternal mortality in Sololá implicitly depended on iyoma referring
their clients to the hospital. Yet, these same iyoma had been spun
out of the global Safe Motherhood Initiative to create a rhetorical
narrative that showcased change and future promise, while culling
them as part of "lessons learned." And this move seriously compromised the ability of Jhpiego or the Ministry of Health to decrease
maternal mortality.

The director of Jhpiego in Sololá undoubtedly saw the shift away
from iyoma with the new funding cycle as problematic. She had
worked hard under the MotherCare contract to build relationships
with the local iyoma and now was asked to essentially ignore those
relationships because they were no longer a funding priority. While
it is quite easy to change policy on paper and write in or write out
actors as need be, it is not so easy to do this when you are a health
worker being asked to establish relationships with people. It is awk-
ward to know that last year you were telling midwives how important they were and attempting to recruit them, and this year
someone is telling you that they are ancillary to your work. As the
spotlight that focused on the importance of midwives went through
continual cycles of brightening and dimming, iyoma were particularly sensitive to being abandoned.[21] For example, they were vo-

cal about how in the past they had been given kits and credentials to practice, but that now no one resupplied their kits. The director of Jhpiego firmly believed that incorporating iyoma into the Safe Motherhood program was an important complementary goal, regardless of what the official policy said.

After two years of concentrating exclusively on emergency obstetric care, she decided to begin working more directly with midwives. Jhpiego and the Ministry of Health had already provided funds for monthly contact between health workers and iyoma, primarily to encourage midwife referrals through continuing education. There was, however, no extra money to develop programs that specifically focused on midwives or further integrated them into the public health system. Nonetheless, convinced that integration was the path toward decreasing maternal mortality, in 2001 Jhpiego's director in Solalá convened a series of department-wide meetings of iyoma. Jhpiego provided money for the iyoma's transport, a snack, and lunch. To keep down costs she asked that each village only send two iyoma. The point of the meetings was to talk to the iyoma about the health system and the best ways to serve women in Solalá in order to decrease maternal mortality. As the meetings went well the director asked the iyoma to consider if they would like to formally start working with the hospital. Together they worked to outline a list of the iyoma's responsibilities for maternity patients in the hospital, the resources that they would need to make the program happen, and how the program would function. The iyoma took ownership of the program design, to the point of making uniforms for each iyom that had her name embroidered on it. The crux of the program to bring the iyoma into the hospital in Solalá consisted of each iyom covering a twenty-four-hour shift in the maternity ward on the same day of the month, every month.

This was not the first time that iyoma had been invited to the Solalá hospital. Maternity ward staff told me about a prior attempt where they built a traditional Mayan sauna outside of the maternity ward, hoping then that iyoma would come and deliver in the hospital.[22] The logic was that saunas were integral to the traditional birthing process, and that if they built one an iyom would feel encouraged to bring her clients to the hospital for their births. If there were problems during the delivery, biomedical staff would be on hand to help solve the problems.

This early intervention is an excellent illustration of the proclivity of the hospital staff to understand birthing in Solalá vis-à-vis using the tropes of traditional and modern. The intervention assumes that indigenous people in Sololá want a "traditional" setting to give birth, so the hospital tried to recreate that setting. Yet the discussion of birth in chapter 2 reveals how this assumption might be a misconstrual. Indigenous families were interested in homebirth precisely because it was at home—the center of the family—not because it was the most traditional location they could find. To explain the lack of success of the sauna intervention, some of the nurses said that the sauna was not built right, while others said that once it was built, there was no budget for wood, so no one could really use it. These explanations of failure, however, elide many of the issues of professional jealousy and mistrust that pervade bringing iyoma into the hospital.

Rather than predicating another program on "build it and they will come," the director of Jhpiego (an MD and hospital insider) engaged the iyoma to develop a program together. The former model of having midwives birth clients using the sauna did not attempt to incorporate midwifery into the public health system, but rather tried to increase the proximity of the iyoma's practice to biomedical professional practice.[23] This newer program explicitly integrated iyoma into the public health system by involving them in the maternity ward practice and calling on them to help improve care. For example, part of the intervention to improve emergency obstetric care encouraged better post-partum care for women on the maternity ward. Women are at risk for hemorrhaging after birth, and yet before the intervention no one was checking hospital clients for bleeding after delivery. This problem was identified after the iyoma had been working on the ward for about a year, and they were called on to track and provide post-partum care.

As was to be expected, the new program for iyoma in the hospital did not work exactly as it was laid out on paper. During the initial phases it was hard to find iyoma to come to the hospital, so many had to double up on shifts. Though iyoma officially should have been able to deliver low-risk patients who preferred their services, this happened infrequently. The program in Sololá also suffered from the common problem of doctors and, particularly, staff resisting the incorporation of the iyoma (Kruske and Barclay 2004). For many of the (particularly less-skilled) hospital staff, inviting iyoma to deliver babies in the hospital was not progress. Iyoma had no formal schooling in their trade and were frequently older women who could not even read. Many of the less-skilled hospital staff worked hard to graduate from high school and go to a two-year professional college to learn their trade. They resented that the hospital administration invited someone with no formal training onto the ward to do their jobs.[24] One outcome of this resentment was that the *iyoma* said that they spent a lot of time in the morning with the patients helping them shower. This makes sense, as helping the patients on the ward with their hygiene is not recognized as a skilled job by the professional and auxiliary nurses. I also informally heard that some maternity staff were upset because they were losing money due to the presence of the iyoma. Many patients and their families in Guatemala tip hospital staff or give them gifts, both to express their appreciation and to ensure good care for the patient.[25] Officially, no one—not midwives, not doctors, not nurses—is supposed to accept payment from patients, but the practice continues. Since the iyoma started to work on the ward, much of this monetary recompense that used to go to the nurses now went to the iyoma.

Despite the fact that they were not completely welcomed by all hospital staff, during their monthly meetings with the director of Jhpiego, iyoma agreed that their work in the hospital was very important. The iyoma continually reiterated that they were there for the patients. Thus, no matter what the difficulty was, no matter the conflict with a staff member, they would keep returning to the maternity ward to fulfill their duties because the patients wanted them and needed them there.

The costs of this midwife program were, in comparison, diminutive; nevertheless, there were no budget categories within Jhpiego's accounting system to pay for it. Since Jhpiego's program was supposed to be carried out in conjunction with the Ministry of Health, all of the Ministry's budget for reproductive health in Sololá was dedicated to the programs that Jhpiego had deemed important—i.e., emergency obstetric care. They, therefore, had no other monies to put toward programs with midwives. Support had to be pieced together here and there. One group paid for the midwives' aprons. The United Nations Mission for the Verification of Human Rights and of Compliance with the Comprehensive Agreement on Human Rights in Guatemala, better known as MINUGUA, covered the midwives' monthly meetings. The director of Jhpiego supported the program by paying the 100 Q that each iyom received to cover food and transport for her monthly shift (a fixed cost of $390 US a month) out of her own pocket for the first few months. The costs then were met by Médicos del Mundo. To make the program sustainable, however, the director of Jhpiego was attempting to get each of the municipalities of Sololá to cover the costs out of their budget. It was a relatively small amount, and the municipalities had shouldered no official role in supporting Safe Motherhood in Sololá. Though this plan was rejected by the mayors in the first rounds of negotiations, the director hoped that in the future they would accede.

Looking at the example of Sololá helps illustrate some of the ways that the spin actually threatens our ability to address maternal mortality. The spin necessitates finding the next best intervention. Yet this shift in agenda threatens a discontinuity from program to program that can be detrimental. These programs ultimately rely on relationships between providers, NGOs, state officials, traditional midwives, and clients who are seeking services. Undercutting the campaign's relationship with any of these stakeholders is short sighted. The particular shift between working with midwives and promoting emergency obstetric care might not have been difficult in a part of the world where women did not rely on traditional midwives (like Honduras, for example; Shiffman and Garcés del Valle 2006). But in the overwhelming number of places where almost all women are delivered by traditional midwives, pretending that one can stop funding work with midwives and still work on safe motherhood is not at all realistic. Indeed, as the example in Sololá demonstrates, midwives remained integral to the Safe Motherhood efforts despite the policy shift. In the fight against maternal mortality in Sololá, shifting the focus to emergency obstetric care may have done more harm than good by both alienating midwives and tying up all of the resources available for programs under one, ineffective agenda. The result is that health workers on the ground who ironically were attempting to push forward a progressive program that had met with some success in other settings (Asowa-Omorodion 1997; Jokhio, Winter, and Cheng 2005; van Roosmalen et al. 2005) were unable to sufficiently influence the larger policy agendas in Sololá.

The Highest Rates in the Nation: Fighting Maternal Mortality in Santa Cruz

When I began this project in 1999, just as the focus of the local Safe Motherhood campaign was shifting toward emergency obstetric care, the director of Ministry of Health office in Sololá told me that he was worried that this intervention would not have any effect. He tried to recruit me, an anthropologist, because the problem that he saw was a cultural one: women preferred to follow their traditions and give birth at home. Even if they had a problem they would not go to the hospital. To get to the bottom of this conundrum, he recommended that I do my study in Santa Cruz, the municipality that had the highest rates of maternal mortality in the entire country in 1998.

The director's line of reasoning is what inspired my first round of interviews with Kaqchikel women in and around Santa Cruz. How did women feel about their births? What did they think about all of the women dying around them? Was birth perceived as dangerous? Were they afraid to give birth? What did they think was the cause of the high rates of maternal mortality?

I was surprised to find that women did not think maternal mortality was actually a very big problem. How could women who lived among the "highest rates of maternal mortality in the country" not be shaken by it? Yet the longer I lived in Santa Cruz, the more I realized that there was a disjuncture between what epidemiological calculations looked like to health personnel, versus what maternal death actually looked like to someone who lived in the village.

Conventions used to express ratios of maternal mortality make the number of women dying on paper seem massive; this perception, however, is not borne out in everyday life. Maternal mortality is expressed as a ratio of the number of maternal deaths per 100,000 live births. In 1998, when the ratios in Santa Cruz were high, there were only 153 live births registered in the entire municipality. Statistically then, the ratio of maternal mortality was 3,268 deaths per 100,000 live births.[26] Yet, what does this astronomical maternal mortality rate look like to the average occupant of the village? In absolute numbers, five women died. And these five women did not die all in one neighborhood. The municipality of Santa Cruz consists of two villages and four *aldeas*, which are smaller towns that do not meet the population requirements to be called a "village." While the entire municipality shares its language and dress, it is very spread out. Indeed, due to the difficult geography, there is no road connecting Santa Cruz, the municipal seat with any of the other villages or aldeas in the municipality. Nor is there any market or school or church, etc. that would necessitate an occupant of one town to visit another—at least not on any regular basis. Occurrences in one aldea are not, therefore, readily apparent in Santa Cruz, the town, or vice versa. The year that the municipality topped the list for maternal deaths, one woman died in the aldea of Pajomel, one in Tzununá, and three in Santa Cruz proper. But even these three deaths in one town might not hold the same sway as the epidemiological data makes them appear to have since they were spread out over the calendar year. The villages in the municipality are agricultural and are, therefore, strongly marked by the cycles of planting and harvesting. These cycles do not match up with the calendar year upon which the statistics are based. It is an artifact of the calendar system that the Ministry of Health lumped all of the deaths into 1998. If they had based these deaths on the harvest cycle, which many people in Santa Cruz used to remember the year, they would not all have fallen together. Furthermore, while the department of Sololá itself has continued to experience some of the highest rates of maternal mortality in Guatemala, the rating of Santa Cruz as a major locus of death has fluctuated. While five of the seventeen registered maternal deaths that occurred in Sololá in 1998 were in Santa Cruz, in 1999 they registered just one maternal death out of the eleven in the department. A year later that number fell to zero of twenty-nine maternal deaths in Sololá. In short, although the rate of maternal mortality in Santa Cruz may look rather frightening from an epidemiological standpoint, for the common person in the village it is all but invisible.

Indeed, my interviews showed that most women did not perceive a problem with maternal mortality in their area. They themselves felt that their births were no more or less risky than those in other villages around Guatemala. For women living in pronatalist communities, where their mothers, aunts, and sisters may have seven or eight kids and twelve or thirteen gestations, birth is seen as a relatively "normal" activity. While the Safe Motherhood campaign centered on identifying the dangers in homebirth, the expectation in the village was that births would go well. This does not mean that women are completely ignorant of the idea that birth is a time where women are vulnerable to casualty. Indeed, they often spoke of birth as a liminal state: a woman begins to give birth and no one knows if she is going to make it. No one knows if she is going to come back. The fact that some women don't make it was also accepted. When asked if they knew a woman that had died from pregnancy-related causes, all but 12 percent of women I interviewed said that they did. Frequently, women would begin to count off the names of numerous neighbors and family members lost over the years. Others would tell detailed stories of how it had happened that a woman had died. The emotion underlying the stories was not fear, but sadness. Women sometimes died during childbirth. It was sad, but it happened.

I was most surprised that not only did women not see a problem, but they perceived their births as comparatively safe. While the Ministry of Health bases its judgments of risk on statistical comparisons across geography in Guatemala, women are making their judgments based on their increased access to biomedical obstetric care across time. Women these days, they asserted, have much safer births than women in the past. In their mothers' era there was no hospital. If you had a problem that the iyom could not solve, that was it. There were no other sources of help. There were no operations. Now, women have access to ultrasounds, x-rays, pharmacists, doctors, and the hospital. If you had a problem, your family could find you help. Indeed, this perspective was upheld by many of the older women who I interviewed. Ricarda told a story of her first baby, which was transverse. She said that she had labored for two days and two nights, but that the baby just didn't come out. She said that the midwife and her family all agreed that she was having a terrible problem and might not come back from this birth. I asked her then why she didn't go to the hospital. At that time, she said, there was no hospital. Before it was not like it is now. Women who have problems now can get help. In the past, she said, women had to suffer alone.

From the perspective of someone living in Santa Cruz, it is difficult to justify devoting one's scarce resources of time and energy to a problem that has actually substantially *improved* over the last decade, while ignoring problems that are even more pervasive than maternal mortality. Over the years that I lived in the village, Cruceños were extremely upset by the fact that their water supply completely disappeared for several weeks of the year. Not having access to any water is a crisis that can create immeasurable death and sickness. Women and their families were also faced with extremely difficult conditions of poverty, violence, and racism. In short, in Santa Cruz it made no sense to prioritize the health of a pregnancy or potential pregnancy over that of one's spouse, children, and in-laws. Yet the Safe Motherhood campaign assumes that they will do just that.

Just like investors who compare and evaluate global health programs to choose the best issues to tackle, women in Sololá evaluate the issue of maternal mortality in relation to other problems in their lives. Certainly, maternal mortality is a problem. If it were their only problem, Cruceños would be terribly worried about it. However, any successful initiative that works on maternal mortality has to recognize and contextualize the problem in relation to the other myriad extreme situations that families in Santa Cruz must face daily.

As Maghboeba Mosavela et al. (2005) point out, community engagement is essential to building a successful health promotion program precisely because the agendas of researchers or health workers can differ so vastly from those of community members. Hopefully the new shift in Safe Motherhood toward a continuum of care has ended the necessity of spinners to maintain the primacy of the problem of pregnancy-related death. Instead, as we saw in the previous section, space and time must be created to allow health workers to consult with communities about the relative role of maternal care in their lives.

Unsafe Motherhood?

How is it that in a little over twenty years, maternal mortality has changed from a sad event generally ignored in political circles, into one of the major global development problems facing us this century? Answering this question involves getting a handle on the spin. If one were to believe the timeline depiction of events, milestones not only serve to mark the passing of time, but for Safe Motherhood are crafted to create a particular momentum. This moment makes us feel that we are closing in on maternal mortality, that we have learned invaluable lessons over the years and, "we know what works" (Freedman et al. 2007; Campbell and Graham 2006). Maternal mortality is complex, and the spin presents a problem with (a few) global solutions that promise to bring relief regardless of context.

The spinning tells us about the verticality of Safe Motherhood, where program designs and funding priorities around the world are decided by how well a cause can court and lure governments and donors into a relationship. Web pages, retrospectives, and reports are all constructed not only for the general public, who might or might not be listening, but to convince donors to continue to fund efforts to decrease maternal mortality. And what is wrong with that?

In this chapter, I have argued that the affects that the spin has on our ability to curb maternal mortality are far-reaching. While the spin itself may form a persuasive narrative, the primary goal of this narrative is to attract investors and convince them that Safe Motherhood (or Making Pregnancy Safer) is a winning program to fund. The spin, therefore, necessarily obscures the most pressing conversations that deserve our attention: How can maternal mortality reliably be estimated? What evidence do we need to be basing our policies on? What sorts of interventions should drive our attempts to decrease maternal mortality? Should we continue to jump in and try new things, or is Safe Motherhood bankrupt until someone can produce a rigorous randomized control trial or accurately evaluate cost-effectiveness?

In Safe Motherhood the spin does not just help direct what donors fund, it misrepresents to make particular approaches appear far more robust than they are. New interventions like investing in emergency obstetric care are promoted as proverbial magic bullets, while less-fundable interventions, like working with midwives, get spun right out of the program. While it is possible to remove midwives from the spin, in a place like Sololá where iyoma are in charge of delivering the vast majority of women, midwives will remain central to the success of any effort to make pregnancy safer.

The only way biased portrayals like the spin in Safe Motherhood appear realistic is by distancing us from any nuanced, empirical account of Safe Motherhood. This distance assumes a fiction where the specific context of maternal mortality is not relevant to addressing it. The example of Guatemala has helped reveal how untrue this assumption actually is. In Guatemala both the push to decrease maternal mortality and the meaning of pregnancy-related death itself have been heavily shaped by the civil war and the inclusion of the issue in the Peace Accords. Poor (Mayan) woman who die pregnancy-related deaths are regarded as a testament to the government's inability to bring its nation into the twenty-first century. As we will see in the next chapter, this formula can be turned on its head: citizens who do not cooperate with the government's attempts to decrease pregnancy-related deaths can also be viewed as saboteurs.

This distance necessitated by the spin also makes it more difficult for attempts to decrease maternal mortality to transform from top-down initiatives into ones that are more inclusively defined. The example of Sololá shows that it is essential to modify our current modus operandi so that those working in the field can innovate and create some of the policy they are responsible for implementing. Moreover, the failure of the Safe Motherhood campaign to engage the populace in Sololá in a discussion about the relative importance of pregnancy-related mortality in their lives is a severe problem and raises serious questions about the legitimacy of the effort. It speaks volumes about the need not only to go back to the drawing board, but, as I advocate for in my conclusion, to make a more inclusive discussion around actually defining the problem.

Chapter 4

THE INDIO BRUTO AND
MODERN GUATEMALAN HEALTHCARE

─────────────

Tuesday afternoon, four relatives (three males and one female) brought Petrona to the emergency room of the San Juan de Rodas Hospital in Sololá, Guatemala, for a birth-related complication. Petrona lived in the same neighborhood as Ramos, one of the auxiliary nurses who worked in the hospital. As Ramos wheeled her into the ER he related her information to the nurse on duty. Two days ago, Petrona's family came to find Ramos in the village because Petrona was not recovering after giving birth. He went to the house, and after seeing her condition Ramos told her family that Petrona had developed a severe post-partum infection and needed to go to the hospital. Still, the family hoped that her infection would clear up on its own, and only today, nine days after the birth, were they seeking him out again for help, asking him to bring her to the hospital.

I wrote down the information as Ramos told it, and then watched as the family entered the obstetric care unit and the nurse requested that they change Petrona into a hospital gown. She was in pain and grimaced as she was forced to move this way and that in order to pull the huipil over her shoulders and put on her hospital gown. Petrona was older, probably in her 40s. Of the women that I had seen come through the ER, she appeared to be one of the poorest. Her clothing, though beautifully embroidered, was faded and old. Her hair was tangled and had leaves and needles threaded through it (perhaps left over from her treatment in the village). She had large gaps between her teeth, the backs of which had rotted away. She whispered to her family as they attended to her.

When the doctor arrived, he requested that her family leave the room. Before starting her exam he asked her questions to establish a case history: "How long ago did you have the baby?" Petrona was quiet and didn't respond. When no answer was forthcoming, he asked the nurse how many days ago she had the baby. The nurse, who like Ramos was indigenous and from the same area as Petrona, responded jokingly, "I don't know. How many days ago?" "Ask her," he replied. The nurse did not want to do it, made almost no effort and then told the doctor that the woman didn't know when the baby was born. The doctor asks how this was possible, and the nurse shrugged her shoulders, basically saying, "Don't ask me." It was 2:12 PM. I flipped back a page in my notebook to the notes I took at 1:57, where I had written down that Ramos told the ER nurse that the baby was born nine days ago. Why would the nurse deny knowing when Petrona gave birth? Why would she tell the doctor that Petrona herself had no idea?

My attempts to answer these questions have inevitably brought me to more closely examine Foucault's writings on the relationship between the State, institutions providing healthcare, and subjectivities. Foucault (1973) provides a persuasive example of how public institutions that care for patients arrange that care to forward a State's ideas about the type of subjects it desires as citizens. Foucault describes how immediately after the French revolution, existing hospitals were dismantled and doctors were eliminated. By ridding France of monarchy, oppression, and hierarchy, the revolutionary State paved the way for a new French citizen who would neither suffer the diseases of poverty (because the poor had been emancipated), nor the diseases of the luxury (because privilege of the upper classes had been removed). Health institutions were purged because the ideal, new State subjects would have no need of them. I build on this insight to understand Petrona's experience in the hospital in Sololá. In this chapter I consider the hospital as a State institution that reflects its agenda to push Guatemala forward into a new, "modern" era.

While the term *modern* has a plethora of referents, I draw on Fredric Jameson's (2002) work in my own use of it. Jameson suggests that the modern has been used to naturalize a narrative about where we were and where we are now, a narrative which is integral to its lay meaning. Modernity, he points out, is contrasted to a state of past constraint. In the context of the hospital, this past constraint can be imagined to be the lack of a functioning medical system (though the lack of an educational system and judicial system are also relevant). The current medical system (as well as the Safe Motherhood campaign) in Guatemala is therefore based on a western one. As Jameson (2002:8) states: "Never mind the fact that all the viable nation-states in the world today have long since been 'modern' in every conceivable sense, from the technological onwards: what is encouraged is the illusion that the West has something no one else possesses—but which they ought to desire for themselves. That mysterious something can then be baptized 'modernity' and described at great length by those who are called upon to sell the product in question." By not using scare quotes around the term modern, I share in Jameson's doubt that there is any real modern beyond imagining and, perhaps, longing.

Only when we read the doctor and nurse's interaction as an attempt to index Petrona's *lack* of modernity can we begin to understand it. Through the doctor and nurse's commentaries, Petrona was easily remade from a suffering mother for whom a neighborhood mobilized to gather resources to find her biomedical care, into a woman unaware of when she gave birth. In denying that Petrona knew when her baby was born, the nurse stressed that though Petrona and she might both be indigenous, they were separated by worlds of difference; differences so great that the nurse could not even begin to understand Petrona or what she said. By not questioning or pushing the nurse's denial, the doctor allowed for the fact that the identity the nurse created for Petrona was a viable one. And it is the creation of this identity that can help us understand why the interaction is acceptable in this setting. Through this interaction the doctor and the nurse implicitly acknowledge that Petrona has reproduced inappropriately. The example presents a powerful picture of how modernity and reproduction are intertwined by the staff to produce a particularly scathing judgment of Petrona. Her apparent inability to recall when she gave birth dehumanizes her; it then becomes hard to imagine Petrona as a productive member of any society, let alone modern, Guatemalan society.

In this chapter, I represent the fictitious identity that was assigned to Petrona through the trope of the *Indio bruto*. Indio bruto is an epithet occasionally used in Guatemala that captures almost every negative stereotype about being indigenous, something like the imagined "welfare queen" in the United States. The Indio bruto is illiterate, backward, dirty, simple, poor, lazy, and stupid. The trope of the Indio bruto works well here because instead of being a marker of race,[1] it has become something else. In the hospital setting, the identity of the Indio bruto has become shorthand for a client that is not taking on their fair share of nation-building. They are a leftover from the past, representing the oppressive, divisive, impoverished, and backward State that Guatemala was. Identifying the Indio bruto is just the first step of the process. What follows, of course, is an attempt to help educate or remake the client into an appropriate, post–civil war subject.

In this analysis, I use the bureaucracy and policies of the Guatemalan Ministry of Health as a proxy for representing the State agenda to forward modernity.[2] In the first part of this chapter I look at what these policies say about who the clients of the contemporary Guatemalan hospital should be. When we look at how policies affect the everyday lives of clients we can see how out of place these policies actually are in a real, Guatemalan hospital. Rather than treating poor and uneducated clients who live in chaos and (frequently) violence, the policies imagine different, and I argue, modern subjects with modern values. When the imaginary subjects fail to materialize, it falls upon the hospital staff to remake those who do use the hospital. In the second part of the chapter I look at how staff try to address the non-modernity they perceive by educating clients. What goes on in the hospital is an attempt to change people, to show them the ways to behave—to transform Guatemala from a violent, chaotic, post-war nation into the modern nation that the health workers want to live in. Here I argue that health workers attempt to remake their clients in an attempt to remake the State. What I saw was desire or even desperation to live in a modern Guatemala that existed beyond the reach of violence and fear. Staff are particularly placed within the landscape of the country: they come into daily contact not only with the poor and disenfranchised who must rely on the low-cost healthcare provided by the government, but with a group they perceive as future generations. Many health workers signed on for such a difficult and, in some cases depressing job, in the hope that they could do something to change their nation. Thus, they struggled to bring order and modernity to the one small corner of Sololá that they control: the hospital.

Cultural Incompetence: Bureaucratic Officialdom and Imaginary Patients

Miriam, age 24 and six-months pregnant, arrived to the hospital after falling down. She and her husband were concerned with the health of their fetus and decided to go to consulta externa to make sure that it was alright. The doctor did an ultrasound and told her that the baby had died a while ago, but that its death was not related to the fall. He asked her to go home and come back in the morning. Miriam's husband was a little miffed because they had already waited several hours this morning, and now they would have to come back and wait again tomorrow. But the doctor said that there was no reason for her to spend the night in the hospital because no one could help Miriam until tomorrow. The couple came back the next day and waited three and a half hours to be seen. Finally, the doctor did an exam and sent the husband to buy some vaginal suppositories that they needed to start labor. Miriam was checked in and sent to the maternity ward.

Over lunch I ran into Miriam's husband. He asked me to explain to him what they were going to do to his wife. I told him that the suppositories were going to start labor and that it would trick her body into having a normal birth. He was concerned about what would happen if she had problems. At the very worst, I said, they could operate on her. He thought for a moment and then asked me if his family would be responsible for what was born. He was afraid that they would be obligated to pay to depose of the remains of the fetus. He himself thought that it was better for the fetus to stay in the hospital, because it was not really a baby and didn't have anything to do with them. I told him that I had no idea what was going to happen to it.

After lunch I asked the ER nurse what would happen with the fetus. She told me that whether or not Miriam's family would have to take the body depended on how the doctor classified it. If it was a miscarriage, then they "bury" the baby in the hospital. If it was stillborn, then they give it to the family. All of this is depended on how far along the gestation was.

When I saw Miriam's husband the next day, he told me that they gave him the fetus. Not knowing what to do with it, his family sent it to the mortuary shop. They had to pay 250 Q to the owner: 150 Q for the baby coffin and 100 Q for completing the municipal paperwork and burying the baby in the Sololá cemetery. He told me that at first he thought that it would just be cheaper to bring the fetus home with him, and dispose of it himself, but there were other, even stiffer costs associated with this choice. "Why spend more money on this?" he asked.

I wasn't surprised at all by Miriam's husband's lack of interest in the fetal tissue. When conducting interviews with women in the village, I had asked if it was more important for the mother or the baby to survive a birth. Respondents fell into three categories: those that thought that it was important that both survive; those that stressed both were important but that if you had to choose, the mother comes first; and those that definitively answered that the mother was most important. Not one person argued for the importance of the baby. In a setting marked by such high rates of perinatal mortality, it is perhaps not surprising that a fetus in utero and newborns are not mourned in the way that older children, adolescents, and adults are mourned when they pass on. Yet the ways that medical policies in the hospital institutionalized life negated these understandings.

Nancy Scheper-Hughes (1992) has powerfully argued for the connection between an impoverished setting and high child mortality on the formation of parental attachment. But, obviously, institutionalizing an acknowledgement of low parental attachment to the fetus paints a picture of Guatemala as a destitute country. It argues for a citizenry whose beliefs stem from their impoverishment. Instead, the government has attempted to institutionalize a more progressive perspective of life, worthy of a more developed country. In the hospital, biological definitions are used to define whether the product of conception is a fetus or a baby. While on paper these may appear to be well-reasoned classifications based on the ability of the baby to survive outside of the womb if it were to receive adequate medical care, in practice the definition is about desire. The medical resources available to keep a fetus alive in Sololá are diminutive. There is no intensive care unit. The choice in definition is about codifying and imagining modernity, not about improving medical practice.

Despite the fact that Miriam's husband did not want the fetus, he never spoke up. He obviously felt that disagreeing with this hospital policy could inherently mark him as the wrong type of person. The hospital's definition conflicted with Miriam's husband's views of the fetus, and this conflict, from the perspective of those staffing the hospital, spoke to his own impoverished background. Changing the regulations to meet the needs or demands of clientele like Miriam's husband would be allowing poverty into the future, instead of relegating it to the past.

While forcing clients to pay for the disposal of unwanted fetuses was an inconvenience, in other sectors structuring the system to meet the needs of a mostly imaginary modern clientele meant that the hospital didn't work. Sometimes it didn't work for the clients. Other times it didn't work for the clients or the healthcare providers. For example, the hospital relied on the use of official names shown on an identity card or birth certificate to register its patients. The official name is associated with an individual, but persons in Santa Cruz are composites of relationships. Accordingly, official names were often meaningless for anyone except the individual themselves and their immediate family. Because of their irrelevance, parents in Santa Cruz sometimes gave each offspring of the same sex identical official names. On paper there was no way to differentiate these children except for age. In the community, however, identity was easily indexed by a well-charted social space and web of relationships. Nicknames were invented, and context was used to pinpoint exactly who you might be talking about.

The conflict between official and local ways of naming heated up when family members, more distant relatives, and friends attempted to find a patient who had been interned. The family member would tell the nurse that he or she was looking for a woman who had been brought in. Frequently, the only information that they would have about that woman was the place that she lived. The nurses then got annoyed that a patient's relative could not know her name, her age, or what her problem was? But to family members, all of the information that the nurse wanted was arcane knowledge; birthdays were not celebrated and official age was not marked. They were not doctors, so how were they supposed to know what the relative's medical problem was? They already told the nurse that the person they are looking for was sick. The situation became uncomfortable as the exasperated nurse would ask how it was that they would come without any information about the patient and expect the staff to be able to find her.

The hospital's decision to rely so heavily on names, even when it was a continual source of conflict with clients, seemed ideological. It was certainly not impossible to look people up by the village that they came from. And while there might have been more patients from the larger cities, the hospital was small enough that there were never hundreds, let alone tens of patients from the same place.

I would argue that the differences in who relied on the official name and who didn't were not random, but said something about the position of the client vis-à-vis the State. After Rosario died and we were all sitting outside of the autopsy room, waiting for the forensic pathologist to arrive, the police came to take a statement on the death. They were particularly concerned about getting the name of the midwife, who conceivably could have been held responsible for the death if the autopsy had shown a different cause. When one of the officers asked what her name was, Rosario's family came up with Maria and then they tossed around suggestions as to whether

it was Saloj or Chumil and said it was something like that, but in
the end they didn't know. The officer accepted that response. He
never took their lack of knowledge as insubordination, but rather
recognized that not knowing the name of the person who was delivering your daughter's baby was completely possible and normal.
As this example shows, official names are needed by the State, and
not using those names allows one to operate outside of the purview
of the State. To those who felt that the success of a nation relied on
the active participation of all sectors of society, people like Rosario's
family, who paid no attention to official names, were not participating in a manner that included them in the new Guatemala. Rather,
they were being divisive.

Not only were some patients difficult to find, but other essential
systems, like making sure that a sick person was seen by the right
doctor, were equally flawed. Fidelia asked me to accompany her to
outpatient care because she had pain in her abdomen and her menstruation was irregular. We got up early in the morning, took a boat,
took a bus, arrived at the hospital by 7:30 AM, and received our
number in line. When her number was called we both went into the
screening room to see the nurse. She asked Fidelia what her problem was and Fidelia told her that she was having abdominal pain
and stopped. I asked Fidelia to tell the nurse about her menstrual
irregularities, and Fidelia said that she was also having strange periods. The nurse then asked Fidelia what she wanted to be seen for.
She said that Fidelia had two different problems that corresponded
to two different doctors and she didn't know which one to send Fidelia to. Fidelia was completely confused and didn't understand at
all what the nurse was talking about. She had been clear in indicat-
ing her pain and that she needed a cure. Only since I had worked
in the hospital and was familiar with the structure did I know that
there was a gynecologist and an internal medicine specialist, and the
nurse was asking if Fidelia wanted to see the gynecologist for the irregular periods, or the internal medicine specialist for the abdominal
pain. Fidelia wanted to be treated for her pain, yet she did not have
the knowledge required to answer the question.[3]

Lack of familiarity with biomedical diagnosis also led to the clients' inability to understand questions that doctors asked. For example, a father brought in his 6-year-old son who was experiencing
acute abdominal pain. When the doctor came over to examine the
child, he put his hand on the child's abdomen and pressed down,
asking if it hurt. He then released the child's abdomen and enquired
again whether it hurt. The father answered that it did. The doctors

told the father that he was not asking him, but rather asking the child. The father replied that the child couldn't understand Spanish. So the doctor asked the father to translate. The doctor pushed down, paused and released. The father again answered that it hurt, but the doctor told him that he needed to know what the child felt, and thus it was important for the father to ask if it hurt when he pressed down or let up. Attempting to be compliant, the father asked the child in Kaqchikel, "Does it hurt when the doctor does that?" and then told the doctor again that, yes, it hurt.

> Doctor: Which? When I press down?
> Father: Yes.

After the interaction, which struck me as strange, I asked the doctor to explain to me what had happened. He told me that there are two different diagnoses for the child's general symptoms, and they are distinguished by when the abdomen hurts. One hurts more when you push down. The other hurts more when you release. I would argue that to understand such distinctions and to find them relevant necessitates a certain understanding of biomedicine, an understanding that is neither present in nor accessible to many of the Ministry of Health's clientele.

One day during a lull in the ER I started a discussion about clients' complaints concerning the care they received at the hospital. The general opinion was that until Guatemala provided a decent education to all of its citizens and literacy was the norm, the complaints would not change. The doctors interpreted the problem as the patients' lack of understanding of biology and biomedicine. Because I had tried to help students in Santa Cruz prepare for a potential college education, I realized how rare biological knowledge was in Guatemala. Biology was not a mandatory course in the Guatemalan school curriculum and only those select few ever had any exposure to the science.

I certainly agreed with the doctors that if the hospital's clients were literate and had a firm knowledge of biology that they would not have so many problems with the hospital (and vice versa). However, I held that position not because of their knowledge per se, but rather because of what such a change in the populace would say about the country. A Guatemala where all citizens were educated to a level that they could read, let alone understand biology, would be an inclusive Guatemala that did not suffer from the harsh divisions that I encountered. The design of the hospital system seemed to preclude rather than to facilitate efficiently attending patients. Yet when asked, doctors found the state of the State—the lack of education, the poverty—unacceptable. They did not readily object to the system, which would work for an educated, yet not-yet-existent clientele. I now turn to look at the problems created for a client who fails to ascribe to the characteristics of the ideal State subject or who is suspected of being an Indio bruto.

Noncompliance

Despite the fact that the official system was geared toward a not-yet-existent clientele, those who could not or would not participate as they were expected to were essentially cut off from care. Noncompliant patients were free to release themselves or refuse care, but in order to do so they had to sign a book of official acts, stating that they were cognizant of their actions, that they were ignoring medical advice, and that they would not hold the hospital liable. I also heard one nurse give a slightly different interpretation of the function of the book to a patient: if you sign it, then the hospital is no longer responsible for treating your problem. In this particular case the point that the nurse wanted to make was that if the patient signed the book, he could not come back. The use of a book of official acts is paramount to the legal structure of the country and reaches into the functioning of every municipality. Most people have to sign a municipal book several times over the course of their lives. In my two years of fieldwork I also had occasion to sign it. The fact that a book is used in the hospital clearly connects this setting to the institutional framework of the State. Though I frequently heard about the book in the hospital, I never actually saw it, nor did I ever hear of anyone signing it.

Patients and their families obviously viewed the book as a threat because in the hospital we frequently talked about patients who "escaped." Silvia's story illustrates how non-compliant patients feel they need to flee the hospital without confronting the staff or signing. Silvia was an extremely friendly and open woman whom I met in the maternity ward after she had been hospitalized for high blood pressure. She married at age 18, and at 29 she had a complicated reproductive history. This was her sixth pregnancy, though she only had three living children. Her fourth pregnancy resulted in a stillborn baby that was birthed at home after six months of gestation. The fifth pregnancy was also stillborn, but it was birthed in the hospital after seven months of gestation. After each of these incidents she was interned in the hospital for eight days and had to undergo a dilation and curettage procedure (D&C).[4]

Silvia knew that she had a chronic problem with high blood pressure, and that blood pressure was the cause of the last two deaths of her babies. She told me that her iyom was also aware that she had high blood pressure, but that the iyom had no idea how to help her. Silvia felt that after so much experience with pregnancy and problematic blood pressure she now knew when she was having problems. First, she got a very strong headache, and then it would turn into a pain in her uterus and the baby would move around a lot. It hurt her to pee because of varicose veins and she could also get pains in her arms, legs, or head. If she had any of these symptoms she would go to the health post to get help.

I talked to Silvia on a Thursday and she related to me the experiences she had had that week. She was about six months pregnant and started to have what she knew were problems with her blood pressure. On Monday morning she got up and went to the health post in her small, rural area to get help. The auxiliary nurse in the health post knew that Silvia's case was complicated and therefore gave her an appointment to see the doctor the next day in Panajachel, the closest health center boasting a doctor. Unfortunately, Silvia could not make it on Tuesday, but Wednesday morning she packed up and took the one and a half hour bus trip to the health post, but the doctor was not there. They told her that she would need to travel farther and go to the health post in Sololá. She took another twenty-minute bus trip and fifteen-minute walk to get to the Sololá health post, where they took her blood pressure. Her pressure was so elevated that they told her she would have to be admitted to the hospital. One of the doctors saved her the thirty-minute additional walk and drove her there.

The gynecologist on call at the hospital explained to me that Silvia would have to stay in the hospital for four to six weeks, being monitored and receiving the medication to control her blood pressure, until they were able to do a c-section. Silvia was not at all happy about the treatment. She asked me how it was possible for her to stay in the hospital for a month and a half. She was completely out of her element. She told me that her husband was an agriculturalist who grew broccoli and eggplant. They had 15 *cuerdas* of land and he had to walk a significant distance every morning.[5] How would her husband work if no one was there to cook for him? But worse yet, who would take care of her three children, one of whom was very small? I asked the doctor if she couldn't go home and have someone else administer the medicine. He told me that she needed medicine at night as well as in the day. The only person with the skill to administer an intravenous shot was the nurse, who first of all was lo-cated a significant walk away from Silvia's house, and second of all did not work in the night or on the weekends. Sending her home was condemning her to not getting the treatment that she needed.

The hospital social worker was called in to handle the question of Silvia's kids. Arrangements were made with the administration that the children would be brought into the hospital to live in the children's ward while their mother convalesced in maternity. That way their basic needs would be provided for and they would not be separated from their mother. Silvia's husband could arrange to eat with a relative while the family was gone.

The arrangement did not suit Silvia at all. She emphasized that bringing her children to the hospital was a bad idea, because the hospital was full of disease and sickness. What sort of place was it for the children to play? Furthermore, she told me again, she could not just sit in a bed for a month and half. It was as if they were asking to her to be in solitary confinement or trying to punish her. She was already "bored," and had only been in the hospital for three days.[6] She was feeling a little better, though, and the doctor said that her blood pressure was responding to the medication.

On Sunday morning when I returned to the ward to do an inter-view with a woman who would be discharged, I could not find Silvia. I asked the nurse about her and was told that yesterday, during visit-ing hours, Doña Silvia had "escaped" from the hospital. She said that they only found out because the women who were Silvia's bed neigh-bors told the staff what had happened. A group of family members had shown up to visit her. Silvia got out of bed, they all surrounded her so that she was hidden, and they walked out of the door together with Silvia in the middle. Theoretically, Silvia was free to leave the hospital at any time; all she had to do was to sign the book. Instead, she escaped—and escaped wearing a rather skimpy hospital gown.

The campaign to decrease maternal mortality was in place to pre-vent pregnancy-related death. Pre-eclampsia, however, could easily develop into eclampsia, which would be fatal. Here was a clear ex-ample of someone who was very seriously at risk. Silvia had been identified by the health system, and referred up the chain. The NGOs and Ministry of Health in Sololá knew about her. Nevertheless, there was no part of medical system that was designed to respond to the needs of women like Silvia. It was just assumed that she would be able to disappear from her home for months at a time.[7]

Sylvia's story also gives us important insight into the book, which is an attempt to officially distinguish those who act in a sanctioned manner from those who refuse to participate in an acceptable way. Many patients escaped from the hospital instead of signing the book— even Silvia, whose doctor recommended a treatment that was nearly impossible for her to follow. People's negative reactions to signing the book did not come from a lack of understanding of the book, but rather stemmed from the fact that they completely understood it; they did not wish to legitimate their status as someone unable to function within the system. If the system was about serving modern clients, what did their inability to comply with the system say about them? They did not want to be maneuvered into a place where they would leave material evidence that could justify the staff's antipathy. On a figurative level, they certainly would not want to promote any imagined connection between themselves and an Indio bruto.

In short, following a doctor's instructions was important to marking one's self as a particular kind of client. Tine Gammeltoft (2007) comes to the same conclusion after talking to the grandmother of a woman who was counseled by doctors in Vietnam to abort her abnormal fetus. Gammeltoft (2007:158) says, "complying with the advice provided by medical doctors can be seen as an act of belonging, an acknowledgement of membership of a national community that is historically rooted in collective fight for freedom and independence. By accepting a prenatal diagnosis, one also turns oneself into a proper citizen—someone who recognizes and appreciates the efforts invested in building the Vietnam of today." The consequences of not complying with medical advice stretch far beyond the walls of the hospital.

Educating the Indio Bruto

Above I discussed how the hospital created discourses around appropriate responses to one's own biological processes that pair up with an idea of modern, post-war subjects. Here I look at how staff interpret these discourses and apply them to patients. Essentially, the discourses provide a guide for labeling clients as Indio bruto or not. While the treatments that people receive are concerned with healthcare, they are also in part concerned with educating clients about modern behavior. The individual motivations of the nurse that governed how Petrona was treated were undoubtedly complex, but I use examples such as this to highlight the institutional conditions that need to be in place to make such interactions normal, or at least acceptable. I euphemistically call these activities "educating," because educating is ostensibly an important component of health-care and disease prevention. Nevertheless, as Paulo Freire (1970) pointed out, education is never neutral. Much of the educating that I saw in the hospital was certainly not geared toward improving health, but rather toward promoting a particular type of modern client. Educating, therefore, involved pointing out ways that clients were deficient and what they need to do to correct those deficiencies. I return here more directly to the Indio bruto, to show how this imaginary character is often used to fill in the details of clients' lives. The rest of this chapter details the skirmishes that occur in the hospital as clients try to get out of being pegged as an Indio bruto, and get access to the care that they want.[8]

Stereotyping the Indio Bruto

One afternoon as I was sitting in the emergency room doing observations, a grandfather and a father brought in a small child who was burned. They laid the child down on one of the examination tables and then the two men began to relate to the doctor the story of how the child came to be injured. The doctor listened and then he started to examine the child. By this point the nurse had come over to the doctor's side to see if she could help. As he examined the burnt child the doctor talked to his audience without looking up. Unfortunately, he said, the culture here was such that babies and children walk behind grownups and no one worries about what is happening with a child until he gets hurts. When he finished the exam the doctor looked up and told the father and grandfather that they had to take better care of their children.

> Doctor: How old is he?
> Father: Seven.
> Doctor: Is he in school?
> Father: No.
> Doctor: He needs to be studying.

After this exchange the doctor weighed the child and said he was underweight. The doctor then wrote out a prescription for the child's pain, gave it to the two men and told them to put the kid in school. The two men left with the child.

What does a burn have to do with schooling? The doctor pinpointed the cause of the burn as a culture of neglect, when he extolled on the unacceptable state of parents who never pay attention to what their small children are doing. He then went on to fill out what he thought this culture of neglect looked like—people who

don't feed their children enough and don't worry about them getting an education. In short, what we have here is a classic case of
the Indio bruto. While the doctor may rely on the trope of the Indio
bruto to understand the situation, it is also apparent that he is trying in his own, and arguably inappropriate, way to improve this
child's life. For him, this means pointing out to the parents that he
is underweight, telling them that their child deserves to be in school
and that they need to be more vigilant so that they can prevent
accidents.

This example illustrates particularly well the complex role of the
Indio bruto and education in the hospital. On the one hand, healthcare staff undoubtedly can engage in an activity akin to racial profiling, where they use their own imaginary stereotypes to fill out
the details of clients' lives and the causes of their maladies. Yet the
healthcare staff's motivations for "educating" are often more complicated—and even contradictory—than attention to race alone might
lead us to believe. In this vignette we can see the doctor attempt to
correct what he sees as the shortcoming of his clients—they don't
feed their child enough, they don't pay enough attention to him,
and they don't send him to school. Unfortunately, however, little
attention is paid to the structural circumstances that might make
it difficult for his clients to actually change any of these situations.
Instead, the doctor conceives of the problems as how his clients'
choose to behave—in ways that don't mesh with his own idea of a
modern Guatemala.

Clothing the Future

The doctor's hope for this child's future exemplifies healthcare staff's
particular concern for children. In almost every recording I have
where a woman is getting wheeled off either for a c-section or to Labor and Delivery, a nurse can be heard calling, "*y la ropita*?" (and the
baby clothes?) to family members. Outside of the hospital it was not
uncommon to see a newborn dressed up in the same clothes as they
are in North America, but in the past when these clothes were un-
available, newborns were wrapped in cloth, a practice still followed
by less-affluent families. The hospital staff, however, demanded a
layette and staff recited a detailed list of essential clothing needed to
dress each newborn. Families that brought cloths in which to wrap
their babies were told that they must provide the layette clothing
instead.

While the request for clothing may seem innocuous, one of my
worst hospital experiences involved this issue. When her contrac-

tions began, Consuelo, a young, pregnant teenager who was about to become a single mother, asked me to go with her and her father to the hospital. Everything went well until we arrived in the labor room on the maternity ward. A midwife and the nurse were both there to get her settled in. It turned out that Consuelo had not brought clothes to dress the baby after the birth, but instead had only a towel to bundle him up. She had planned to put him directly into her *peraj*, a heavy, hand-woven cloth that women use to tie the babies to their backs. The midwife was explaining to Consuelo's father that he would need to go to the market to get baby clothes. She was detailing for him each of the pieces that he would need to buy. He looked distraught, probably because it was a long and difficult-to-remember list that foreshadowed a high cost. At some point in this negotiation, the nurse interrupted. Speaking only to the midwife, she looked directly at Consuelo's father and said, "*Éste nunca va a saber comprar ropa*," figuratively meaning: This one is never going to be able to figure it out.

As she insulted the man, she never took her eyes off of him. She then transferred her gaze to the midwife and said that she didn't understand why people came to the hospital without baby clothes. She felt that this was not acceptable and that people who show up without baby clothes should just be sent back to where they came from. She would not make eye contact with me, though I was standing right next to her and staring at her. She pretended that she and the midwife were the only people in the room. From my perspective she was being very aggressive. I began to doubt if it was a good idea to bring Consuelo to the hospital and leave her all alone with a nurse that was already angry with her, especially since this was Consuelo's first baby.

Though in my experience this nurse's behavior was quite extreme, it highlights the hospital's attempt to normalize baby clothes over options that might have been more available to poor people, such as hand-woven cloths and towels. It is difficult to justify this preference on medical grounds, and is much easier to understand the nurse's reaction when contextualizing it in respect to the story of the Indio bruto. Her idea of a respectable, responsible patient was someone who used baby clothes. A responsible patient did not show up empty handed to have a baby and expect the hospital to pay for the clothes. While Consuelo had not intended to abrogate this responsibility, the fact that she had brought a towel and cloth to wrap the baby was not only denigrated, but later ignored. It did not matter that she brought cloth, it only mattered that she did not bring baby clothes. The nurse referred to "these people," in one fell swoop defining herself and the midwife in another category, and firmly establishing Consuelo's category as one that was not worthy of care. Importantly, guaranteed healthcare is the birthright of all Guatemalan citizens. In effect, then, the nurse was clearly pushing Consuelo out of those who formed part of the new nation.

Yet this example perhaps speaks most loudly to the fact that as Guatemala moves into the twenty-first century, blood and ethnicity no longer define one's belonging, or lack of it. While the mothers may belong to a disenfranchised generation and their practices denigrated, the babies are not rejected out of turn. They come into the world unsullied, full of potential to assimilate into a modern nation. We can see that new babies are embraced and hospital staff hopes that they will become more assimilated when clothed in the layette of the modern subject. Indeed, there is an importance of treating them like they are part of the future—i.e., making sure that they have the proper clothes to be proper citizens.

Just on Time

In the institutional context of the hospital in Sololá, time took on a particular meaning and clients were alerted to fact that time functioned in an institutionally particular way when they arrived to the hospital gates. The gates were opened to clients seeking outpatient care at 7:00 AM. After a few hours, no more numbers were handed out for a turn to see a doctor. Gates were then closed and the crowds grew as visiting time neared. Once again people flooded the hospital and then were ejected as visiting hours ended. Patients in the hospital also followed a time-bound regimen. Each of their meals was scheduled, as were visits by their family and doctors.

While patients had no control over any of these time-bound activities, they were called on to talk about the timing of their own sicknesses. Clients were certainly aware that the medical professionals in the hospital adjusted and adjudicated the treatments that they would receive depending on the timing of a sickness. Clients were, therefore, put into a difficult position of trying to make the right statements about time to obtain the treatments that they wanted. While it might seem that the timing of the condition is quite neutral or factual, in the hospital in Sololá it seemed anything but. By saying the wrong thing, one could easily slip out of the category of someone deserving of care and into the category of an Indio bruto.

Take, for instance, the following example: a young man came to the hospital saying that he was in pain and had had an accident.

When the nurse asked him when the accident occurred, he said "yesterday." When the doctor later asked, the man said "last night." The X-ray showed that he had a broken clavicle, but it was obvious to the doctor that the injury was much more than twenty-four hours old. The doctor confronted the patient and, pointing at the X-ray, told him that the accident happened a long time ago. The patient just stared at him. The doctor repeated his assertion one more time, but when the patient failed to react the doctor left. The nurse then went to the bay and asked the patient when the accident happened. The patient answered that it happened yesterday, and the nurse responded, "Are you sure?" She then asked him to tell the truth.

Nurse: Look, we are not the police. Tell us the truth.

He told her that the accident happened two nights ago, but the doctor's interpretation of the X-ray indicated that it occurred even longer in the past. The nurse told him that the doctor needed to know when the accident happened in order to treat him. The man continued to insist that it had only just occurred.[9]

By delaying his trip to the hospital after his collarbone broke, the client immediately opened himself up to speculation about his own brutishness. Couldn't he feel the pain? Why didn't he care enough about himself to go the hospital? Was he just apathetic? The client was obviously aware that his delay in seeking treatment would not be acceptable to the health staff in the emergency room, so he tried to avoid their judgments by lying about the timing of the accident. Nevertheless, this dug him in even deeper. Not only did he lie, but he then stopped talking and refused to answer questions. In their eyes he became stubborn and intransigent, if not stupid.

Clients knew that the healthcare staff in the hospital had very specific ideas about when one needed to go to the hospital to seek care. It was particularly important to the staff that there be no delay between an incidence and when a client sought help. Obviously, as discussed earlier, this was imperative in the Safe Motherhood campaign that gave very strict guidelines concerning standardized timing of obstetric events: no more than twenty-four hours in labor, no more than thirty minutes post-partum pushing the placenta, etc. Following these guidelines about time very much separated the modern, responsible patients deserving of care from the *Indios brutos*.

The idea that particular treatments had to be justified by the proper timing was also difficult for clients to navigate. As the following example illustrates clients were not always so clear on what the

"correct" timing was. In the incident I describe below a mother and
midwife attempted to second-guess the hospital staff, and fabricate
what they believed was the appropriate timing (and symptoms) for
the treatment that they wanted for Elena, a laboring young woman.
Though it was obvious that the two women understood the importance of time to the staff, they found the logic on which the importance of time was based very confusing, and thus ended up putting
forward their best guess as to the "proper" timing to get an IV, but
not to risk an operation.[10]

Elena went into labor in the night with her first child, but by the
next day nothing was really happening and the midwife thought
that perhaps this was not going to be a normal, vaginal homebirth.
Four male relatives, two female relatives, and the midwife transported Elena to the hospital, where they took her to the ER. The
nurse gave Elena's mother and the midwife a hospital gown and
asked them to change her. While changing her they started to discuss the delivery. "Maybe the doctor's exam will show that she's
normal," the midwife mentioned. After they finished changing her,
the midwife asked the mother:

> Midwife: What time should we tell them that she started to have
> problems?
>
> Mother: I would say that her labor started yesterday at about 4:00 and
> then the contractions got stronger.
>
> Midwife: Look, they are not going to ask what time she started labor
> yesterday. That really doesn't interest them.
>
> Mother: No?
>
> Midwife: Maybe it would be better to tell them it started earlier. I
> don't know. I can't figure out what we should tell them.
>
> Mother: Yeah. ... We could tell them the same thing that we told
> them last time, not too early but not too late either.
>
> Midwife: About 2:00 in the morning, then?
>
> Mother: Yes. ... That sounds good. Yes ... that's fine.
>
> Midwife: If we tell them it started at 4:00, they won't pay any atten-
> tion to her.
>
> Mother: Yes, I think that saying 2:00 in the morning is better.
>
> Midwife: Yeah, that's better.
>
> Mother: Yeah.
>
> Midwife: And now her contractions have become stronger.

Mother: I would say that she looked like she was going to have the baby at home, and then we came here. Isn't that true? It just seems like she shouldn't take too much longer. The problem is that her body is too tired now. What sort of cure do you think that they can give her? I mean, they might have to do a caesarean.

Midwife: Maybe not. Maybe they will just give her an IV and that will cure her. So let's tell them that she doesn't have very strong contractions or that they are not constant.

Mother: There are periods that she has a few contractions in a row and then other times where she is completely relaxed. ... Maybe then they will give her an IV.

When the doctor entered, the midwife delivered the rehearsed lines:

Doctor: When did her contractions start?

Nurse: Her contractions, doctor?

Midwife: At 2:00 in the morning.

Doctor: Okay.

Midwife: And she has really strong contractions, but just for a few minutes, and then they go away.

Doctor: Okay.

After the exam was over and the nurse had taken the patient's vitals, the midwife was left alone with Elena. She tried to reassure her that everything would be okay. She then coached her on what to tell the doctors.

Midwife: Maybe they are still going to come and talk to you. They are going to ask you what happened. Yesterday you started with your contractions. It is definitely time for you to have the baby, but tell them that there are moments when the contractions are gone and you are relaxed, and other moments when the contractions are very strong. Tell them that sometimes the contractions are very strong and that sometimes they just disappear.

Elena: Okay.

To make sense of Elena's story I have to return to a question that started this chapter: In what sort of institutional context would this type of behavior make sense? Why would Elena's mother and her midwife completely create a new story about the timing of Elena's labor? This example reveals significant ways in which the hospital is not a neutral zone. Elena's family are worried as soon as they walk in that the staff "won't pay any attention to her" and that they will not be able to get the treatments that they want (Berry 2008). Their own feelings of a lack of power in the hospital setting certainly are not only reflective of their position as clients, but also their wider social position. The unspoken question that is always lurking in the background is: are they Indio bruto or are they modern Guatemalans? Can they mark themselves as the type of people who deserve the attention and care that they feel that they need for Elena? Much of obtaining that attention and care comes down to saying the right things. In this particular context they are forced to guess about what the proper timing of Elena's labor may be.

Remaking the State through the Hospital

The skirmishes that occur daily in the hospital speak loudly to the actual divisions that exist between the hospital and the clientele that the hospital serves. The extension of health services to the populace at large has been a focus of government in post–civil war Guatemala. As I have argued in this chapter, however, the ways that the delivery of services has been institutionalized imagines a certain type of clientele. The Ministry of Health is there to serve a modern population, one that is assumed to be bureaucratically literate, Spanish-speaking, have an understanding of biomedicine, and be compliant with it. As I have pointed out in this chapter, however, these desires are emphasized over the populace's own actual abilities and needs.

I invoke the specter of the Indio bruto to help illustrate the struggle of self-definition that occurs in medical settings. While many clients do not have the skills they need to navigate the system, they struggle to distinguish their own poverty and lack of knowledge from a lack of interest or agency. However, sometimes one's attempts to collaborate fall flat. For its part, the staff is frequently engaged in education campaigns that often end up negating patients' dignity and do the work of setting staff apart from the poverty and ignorance they perceive patients display. The specter of the Indio bruto also gives the Ministry of Health a good excuse for why they are not successful. The services are not set up to and cannot reach people who are, in some sense, beyond help.

Returning to Foucault's example of healthcare in post-revolutionary France helps highlight the perversity of health systems that are designed to meet the needs of imaginary, desired subjects, rather than the actual citizenry. While the social fabric of France may have changed substantially with the revolution, the new, "healthy" State subjects failed to materialize. Sickness and death rose in the wake of the revolution as no healthcare was available. Likewise in Guatemala, redesigning the State from the top down will not be an effective way to meet the health needs of the population. Jonathan Nathaniel Maupin's (2009) research into post civil-war health system reform in Guatemala helps make this point again. As part of the Accords, the State adopted a neoliberally engineered plan to extend healthcare coverage by relying on NGOs to deliver care. Decentralizing and democratizing healthcare in Guatemala is, not surprisingly, a State ideal. Yet the institutional capacity of NGOs to provide effective care is not, currently, existent.

The expectations that the hospital harbors about its patients creates a context of healthcare delivery that, as frequently demonstrated in the examples above, is not necessarily pleasant for its users. This context is yet another example of how the campaign to decrease maternal mortality is affected by elements outside the bounds of the policies themselves. Many families might intentionally wait to bring their daughters or wives to the hospital, knowing that once arrived they may be scolded for being inadequate in a variety of ways. Laboring women might fear having to struggle to define themselves on top of dealing with an obstetric emergency. This crucial break in understanding between patients, their families, and staff undoubtedly takes its toll on women's likelihood to be referred from the village to the hospital. In the next chapter, I further explore how the wider context of violence makes taking women to the hospital additionally menacing.

Chapter 5

EVERYDAY VIOLENCE

FROM A KAQCHIKEL VILLAGE TO THE NATION AND BACK

––––––––––

At the end of the second decade of Safe Motherhood, a number of international organizations joined together to sponsor the third conference on maternal mortality. The agendas of the past conferences in Nairobi and Sri Lanka focused on strategies and interventions to reduce maternal mortality. The Women Deliver conference, however, tried a different tack (Gill, Pande, and Molhotra 2007; 2007:196). The premise of the conference was that we already understood how to decrease maternal mortality—increase funding to maternal healthcare (including prenatal care, skilled attendance, and emergency obstetrics). What was lacking was the political will from donors and governments to invest. Yet healthy mothers were paramount to the social and economic development of countries. As the conference slogan put it, "Invest in women—it pays."

I have mixed reactions to the Women Deliver strategy. I am heartened by the push from core international agencies to link the problem of maternal mortality to women's connections with their families, their leadership roles, their income-generating power, and their general empowerment. Yet at the same time I am left feeling lukewarm by the basic subtext of the conference: governments and funding agencies (which are arguably male dominated) undervalue women.[1] The premise is problematic in that it groups all women together by assuming a common problem (they are undervalued) and a common solution (investing in women's healthcare). But more disturbingly, it creates a counter-narrative that precludes a deeper understanding of the common everyday challenges that poor women *and men* both face.[2]

What are poor people's everyday challenges? And how do these common challenges impact the ability of the international community to make pregnancy and birth safer?[3] This chapter approaches these questions ethnographically by exploring how violence, a particularly insidious challenge faced by poor across the world, impacts decision-making related to birth.

Writing about violence for an audience accustomed to stylized violence can present particular problems. The reader cannot know about violence in Guatemala unless I first describe it. But the reader may be so inured to descriptions of violence that the purpose of describing is lost. It is impossible to understand the impact of violence on the lives of indigenous and poor if that violence is objectified, or turned into a thing to be viewed or watched, what Valentine Daniel (1996:4) describes as a "pornography of violence." For a viewer (or reader) to dispassionately watch means that she feels immune to danger. But violence impacts on the lives of the poor precisely because it creates a space of potential horror where no one is immune.

To move beyond a pornography of violence I want to imbue the reader with a sense of how disorienting extreme violence can be in one's everyday life. The uncertainty that violence creates makes the seemingly logical become illogical, and can make the absurd stand in for the real (Taussig 1984). My own experience was that I had to learn to think twice about things that until that time had seemed rote—like getting up to answer the door because someone knocked. I use a style here which deliberately tries to overwhelm so the reader not only learns about some of the everyday challenges faced by some Guatemalans, but also, in some way, experiences how disorienting it may be.

The impending possibility of potential horror means that for poor, indigenous Guatemalans, "fear [i]s a way of life" (Green 1994). The origin of that fear for this era of history is relations between the Maya majority and the Guatemalan State, which entrenched the exploitation of "state against nation" (Trouillot 1990). I begin my discussion with colonization to emphasize the point that the legacy of violence in Guatemala has deep historical roots, and despite the end of the most recent civil war, continues onto this day. Poor in Guatemala are the victims of "everyday violence" (Scheper-Hughes 1992)—there is no peace-time protection for them.

Perhaps one of the most insidious aspects of violence in Guatemala is that there is little separation between the exploited and exploiters; those who might be exploited in one situation exploit in another. How can we understand this? Why do those who suffer so much not identify with each other? On the one hand, Scheper-Hughes (1992), who tackles the same question across different domains, bases her explanation in the class antagonism that so heavily marks the Brazilian context. She draws on Gramsci and Freire to show how the poor of Bom Jesus get embroiled in the discourses that suit the interests of the middle and elite classes, causing them to collude in their own oppression. Collusion is and has certainly been present in Guatemala. For example, during the civil war indigenous villagers organized and patrolled their own villages at the behest of the army.[4] Similar to the poor of Bom Jesus, ex-military generals and other right-wing candidates that promise a strong-handed approach against crime can also be popular with poor in Guatemala. On the other hand, Linda Green (1994) shows us how violence can beget mistrust and fear, which operate apart from discourses concerning class. As Green (227) describes it, fear in Guatemala is not "an acute reaction[,] it is a chronic condition." Constant fear creates uncertainty that rips communities apart—it is impossible to tell truth from gossip, friend from enemy, safety from danger.[5] Fear, in short, erases any sympathy or trust that one might assume should reside with a neighbor. While a legacy of violence creates a blueprint of what to do, fear creates the context that justifies a preemptive strike or revenge.

To answer the question of how a constant threat of violence affects decision-making related to birth, I highlight how two different domains—the historical and the present day—blend. It is difficult to identify the marks of violence, both permanent and impermanent, on citizens in Santa Cruz without digging into the ill of a nation, a history of marginalization, war, and disrepair. Only when thoroughly steeped in the legacy that has created the Guatemala that one steps into today, do the daily challenges that make people weary of seeking emergency obstetric care come to life.

Violence and Writing about Guatemala

When I first decided to do research in Guatemala I looked for key readings that might help me understand important characteristics of the country. One scholar of indigenous Mexico, whose advice I sought, divided books into those that concentrated on the constant,

unrelenting pillaging and abuse of Indians, and those that also included other points. That someone would suggest one of the dominant scholarly genres in writing about Guatemala has been centered
on violence and abuse of indigenous people clearly makes a point
about the unusual extremity and prevalence of violence in this setting. My colleague's advice was to get a healthy dose of injustices,
and then, when I am depressed and almost despondent, start reading some of the other stuff. All of the abuse is true and must be documented, but as an approach to scholarship, he argued, the genre
was not going anywhere else. After years of reflecting on his contention I have reluctantly come to agree with him.

I tell this story because I want to highlight how difficult it is to
write about a setting that has been characterized by extreme oppression and at times by genocide against indigenous Maya. My major
challenge is how to provide an adequate description of what people
have lived through over the last five hundred years without elid-
ing that experience, and still write a book that is ostensibly about
something else. I do not want to add to the injustice by short-shrift-
ing this important aspect of Guatemalan history, yet space is too
dear to even hit all of the major points. I am, therefore, going to
limit myself to talking about what I think are the most influential
events that help us understand the level of violence that people live
through today.

The seeds of the current political, economic, and social problems
were sowed when a group of Spanish nobles and notables arrived in
the 1500s to claim their fortunes from the territory that we call Guatemala.[6] But how were they supposed to make money with no gold
or silver to mine? Essentially, they had to squeeze value out of the
one resource that they did have: indigenous communities. The Spanish Crown created a system of *repartamiento*, where subjects were
granted rights not only to the few tracts of arable land, but also dominion over indigenous communities, including the right to tax and
the right to the labor of Indians. From the inception of the colony,
the ability of the colonizers to make money depended in part on the
movement of Indian conscripts from their villages to agricultural
plantations to provide slave labor for at least part of the year.

Many vestiges of this early political/economic system reach into
current Guatemala. The repartamiento began the institutionalization
of labor migration. Even as forced conscription has ended, many of
the poorest indigenous Maya continue to farm plots of corn and
beans in their villages during one part of the year and then migrate
to plantations to earn cash during another part of the year. The re-

partamiento system also created a relationship between indigenous and the State that revolved around extraction—metaphorically, the communities were the mines, and the State tried to pick at them and take out as much value as possible without causing them to collapse. The metaphor of mining vividly captures the idea that the State's extraction of ore from within the indigenous communities has been violent.

The repartamiento system also began the differentiation of class and ethnic groups in Guatemala. The Spanish Crown would only grant labor and land rights to Spanish citizens born on Spanish soil, creating within Guatemala landless children of Europeans, who needed to find creative ways to make their own fortunes. It also designated a group of persons who were of mixed heritage, called *ladinos*.[7] The Crown attempted to protect its labor pool from landless groups by restricting the movements of non-Indians in Indian villages. While many have assumed that this was the making of modern ethnicity in Guatemala, Carol A. Smith (1990a) argues that these differences were meaningfully reinscribed in the late 1800s when the economic focus shifted to coffee. The elite needed an extensive labor pool to make their plantations viable. Up until that time, Smith argues, there was little status difference between non-European groups (e.g., indigenous and ladino). However, the State and the landed elite colluded to coerce the indigenous population into providing labor. The ladinos became the middle men, labor recruiters, and administrators of the system.[8] It is at this moment that the ladinos acquire more status than indigenous, reflecting ideas of the elite's race hierarchy. Smith pegs the rise of the "Indian problem" to this period.

What is the "Indian problem"? Like many other nations, Guatemala has to contend with an incredibly diverse population as it struggles to become a "whole, homogenous and functioning 'modern nation'" (Nelson 1999:2). In Guatemala, power and resources lie in the hands of the ladino ethnic group, who are confronted by the "problem" of dealing with the vast indigenous population.[9] Approaches to the "Indian problem" have shifted over time.[10]

The later half of the twentieth century marked one of the most protracted periods of ladino State-perpetrated violence aimed at controlling and even eliminating indigenous communities. Civil strife in Guatemala ramped up in the beginning of the 1960s, culminating in a full-fledged civil war involving a government-sponsored genocide against the indigenous population in the 1980s.[11] The story of Rigoberta Menchu focused international attention on the shocking brutality with which the Guatemalan army treated its citizens

(Menchu and Burgos-Debray 1984). The Commission on Historical Clarification (CEH) (1999), who was charged with the mandate of documenting what exactly happened during *La Violencia*, as the civil war is also called, outlines how the government publically rationalized its violence against the population by claiming to protect the country against the imminent threat of communism posed by guerrillas. Translated, this meant that many individuals who were perceived to have power to organize—student, health worker, community leader, human rights activist, academic, member of a farming cooperative, etc.—were murdered.[12] The army also considered the indigenous Mayans to be "natural allies of the guerillas." During the height of the violence the army began an aggressive scorched-earth policy, where if they found any evidence of guerrilla support in a town or village, they would simply rape, pillage, and murder to destroy the town.[13] This policy led to the wholesale "extermination of many Mayan communities," eliminating not only the civilian population, but also "their homes, cattle, crops and other elements essential to survival."[14] Evidence has been collected of 626 such massacres. In total, the CEH estimates that 83 percent of the victims of the war were Mayan, and in 93 percent of the cases the State was the perpetrator of violence. It estimates that over 200,000 people were killed and over 1,000,000 people displaced.

In 1996 the Peace Accords were signed, ending both the civil war and the era of overtly solving the "Indian problem" through State-sponsored terror. The Peace Accords consist of a number of agreements on problematic areas including human rights, indigenous identity, and constitutional reforms, as well as a ceasefire agreement. What I find most valuable about the documents is the clear narrative defining the national problem and the solution. The problem is that Guatemala's "social, economic, cultural and political development [have been] impeded and distorted" by the unrest and instability caused by "poverty, extreme poverty, discrimination and social and political marginalization" (CEH 1999). The solution to Guatemala's underdevelopment, as carved out by the Accords, lies in eradicating the social inequities that so severely mark the nation.

For my purposes, I want to highlight two important aspects of the Peace Accords. First, they radically transform the State's relationship to Guatemala's indigenous peoples; the government has become "an efficient tool of development policies" and the indigenous populace its clients. For example, reducing maternal mortality by 50 percent by the year 2000 is an example of a goal laid out in the Peace Accords. As I argued in chapter 3, while this may seem like a neutral goal, in practice the vast majority of pregnancy-related death and sickness in Guatemala is confined to indigenous mothers who are poor, have no formal education, and are unemployed (MSPAS 2003). Again, we must note the striking overlap between the individuals classed as at risk for a maternal death and those who the government victimized during La Violencia.

Second, the Accords constantly invoke the importance of participation of all sectors of society—read indigenous people. The president's own report on how his administration would implement the Peace Accords has a telling subtitle: "Together we Have the Opportunity to Transform Guatemala: Let's Go Toward Change!" (Presidencia de la Republica de Guatemala y Secretaria General de Planificacion 1996). I agree with the tenor of the Accords that active participation from all sectors of society is undoubtedly paramount to a healthy democracy. Yet I will argue that the document on the one hand sanctifies a multiethnic nation that accommodates different creeds and languages, while on the other makes this concession meaningless by proscribing a certain type of participation. This type of participation, of which using the hospital for birthing is representative, essentially asks indigenous Maya to relinquish whatever bits of autonomy that they have struggled to maintain or regain over the last five hundred years.[15] But is this a reasonable request? How does a State that once preyed upon its population then become its primary benefactor? Can institutions, like the State, really transform from hostile to benevolent with the stroke of a pen? The levels of everyday violence and exploitation that were rife while I lived in Santa Cruz La Laguna, and during my travels around Guatemala, made me understand why people would not trust State institutions, and, accordingly, not "participate" in the post-civil war State. In other words, the violence past and present in Guatemala frequently made the option of seeking obstetric care in a State hospital appear to be a bad idea.

Justice, Government, or a Lack Thereof

During fieldwork, the seemingly innocent refrain "En Guatemala, todo es posible" (In Guatemala, anything is possible) eventually sent shivers down my spine. For me the saying encapsulates the absence and failure of government that I witnessed. In Guatemala everything *is* possible because there are no hard and fast rules that everyone plays by. While this creates an unusual amount of opportunity for the entrepreneurial, it also reminds me that what appears quotidian can become dangerous. Tides can turn in one minute. Justice that may have been denied for decades or centuries may be demanded or extracted within the blink of an eye. The crisis of justice that pervades people's lives is closely tied to the incredible prevalence of violence (and crime) and the complete inability of the State to do anything about it.

My first summer in Guatemala was spent in the Petén, where there was a rise in the number of people reported to have had their throats slit in the nearby market in Santa Elena. The attacks were, supposedly, muggings, and the punch line of these stories always pertained to how much money the mugger had stolen. Slitting someone's throat who had, say 100 Q (three- to four-day's salary for a day laborer) was completely reasonable, where killing someone who only had 10 Q (less than half a day's salary) was senseless. Over and over again, people claimed, it just showed how cheap life had become. Indeed, one need only read the newspaper headlines to find out what Guatemalans considered to be a pathetically low price for life: "Clerk Killed for 15 Q"; "Street Vendor Shot for 10 Q."

As people attempt to make meaning out of so much death and so much violence, they look for reasons why it wouldn't happen to them. "What do you expect when you take 100 Q to the market?" people would ask. Reckless behavior like that will get your throat slit. No one, however, points out that taking 100 Q to the market is not a behavior limited to the rich as the rich use grocery stores, and as a *quintal*—the 100 lb bag of corn that is a staple in any poor family's kitchen—may cost about 100 Q during certain times of the year. These stories buck the Robin Hood narrative: the poor are supposed to steal from the rich. What sort of world is it when the poor steal from the poor, people ask? What is the point in that?

The crisis in justice is evident in the fact that protection from the ravages of violence has become an industry. In the mornings when I had to stay in the city to visit the central offices of the Ministry of Health or the university's library, I would hit the streets for the 7:00 AM commute. Rather than seeing men leaving their houses with lunch pails and briefcases, men would be walking to work with their sawed-off shotguns or semi-automatic weapons propped on their shoulders. In fact, there were armed guards everywhere in the city—not just in the restaurants, but in book stores and ice cream parlors. In Zona 9, where the young and wealthy in Guatemala City go out at night, and where some of the more expensive hotels are located, armed military men were posted on every street corner, every night. Some banks had the revolving iron gates that I have seen protecting the subway exits in New York City. You can get in, but once in, don't assume that you are going to make a fast escape.

There is no doubt that the poor in Guatemala pay most for the violence. On the way to a meeting in the city one morning a woman boarded the bus and sat next to me. Since it was a holiday the rest of the bus was virtually empty. After a moment she struck up a conversation. I asked her why she was out on a holiday and she told me that she had to go and identify the body of her son. Apparently, he had been shot to death two days earlier. The police potentially identified the body and had called her that morning to come to the morgue for the final ID. Because it was a holiday it had taken her three hours to get to there. She saw the body and it was her son. The police told her that he was better off dead. Even though her son was a *victim* of violence, they alleged that he was part of a gang, i.e., a perpetrator of violence himself. She had to leave him there. She then had to turn around and take another three-hour trip home, changing buses several times. I told her that I was sorry. She told me how terrible the violence was in Guatemala.

It is difficult to believe that the world does not stop because someone's child dies, but it is even more difficult to imagine having to go through the motions that she was going through. Being forced to scrape together money for a bus fare. Sitting there on the side of the road, alone, waiting for hours for each bus to come. Being in limbo for that time, not knowing whether her son was dead or whether this was a case of mistaken identity. Viewing her son's body surrounded by the police who considered him better off dead. Taking that image home with her over another three hours of waiting.

The reaction of the police highlights part of the crisis in justice; urban gangs are blamed for much of the rash of violence. And while this seems like a plausible explanation for newspaper reports of anonymous snipers shooting into passing buses carrying people home from work, it does little to help us understand why over 2,200 women have been brutally murdered in Guatemala since 2001. Amnesty International has outlined its concerns in two different reports (Amnesty International 2005, 2006). The murder rate of women has increased four-fold since the dawn of the millennium, and although men are murdered more frequently, women are far more likely to be tortured, particularly sexually tortured, before being killed. Bodies of women cut apart, strangled, burned, carved with words, or with their nails removed appear abandoned in gutters or on the side of the road. But perhaps the crisis in justice is best illustrated not by the alarming brutality and unacceptable number of deaths, but rather by the fact that, so far, police have only prosecuted *two* cases. The Amnesty report is full of sad and disturbing testimonies of parents recounting their desperation in trying to convince police to look for abducted daughters, only to have the girls' tortured bodies appear the next day. A common theme to the lack of police response is that these disappeared and murdered women had it coming—they were mixed up with gangs or drugs, and, therefore, brought the trouble on themselves. Amnesty International offers a counter-narrative that connects the murder rate to a failed decommission process after the Peace Accords.[16] The torture that these murdered women have been subjected to is uncannily similar to that reported during La Violencia, where 25 percent of victims were women. Guatemalan society has reabsorbed those who perpetrated these crimes. Is it so far fetched to consider the soaring rates of violence against women as connected to the civil war?

Angelina Snodgrass Godoy (2002) argues that we need to think critically about the lasting effects of the violence of the civil war. She uses the example of lynching to show how La Violencia has qualitatively transformed practices. Just as murder rates of women have increased during the first six years after the Peace Accords were signed, the United Nations Verification Mission in Guatemala (more popularly called MINUGUA) recorded an average of over seven lynchings a month. Godoy links rises in this form of human rights violations (or justice, depending on your point of view) to the State's intentional dismantling of local indigenous arbitration systems and the systematic killing of indigenous leaders during the civil war. Army-directed initiatives, such as military justice and organized civilian patrols, filled the void left by eradicating local, traditional systems. People learned and participated in these "new" systems of justice, so that when the army eventually withdrew, victims of State violence became the perpetrators of new violence. For example, Godoy points out that the popularity of burning as an army tactic has now seeped into the popular mind, as evidenced by the fact that lighting someone on fire is the number one means of lynching today in Guatemala.

Godoy's and Amnesty International's point that the civil war might have some lasting relationship to how and why these women are being killed is well taken. There are, however, notable continuities concerning the impunity and the violence with which (particularly poor) women are murdered in Guatemala. Writing on judicial cases in the mid 1900s, Cindy Forster (1999) describes a particularly disturbing story of a body of a woman in indigenous clothing being cast aside on a path traveled by thousands of migrants making their way to coffee plantations for the harvest. She had not only been decapitated, but the police described her body being attacked by vultures in their report. Nevertheless, there was never any investigation into the death, nor were there any attempts made to join the body with its head. Case descriptions such as this one prompt Forster (56) to ask: "Why did officials charged with preserving peace believe there was nothing strange in acts of violence against women, especially Indian women? And how did the women and men involved both share and sometimes challenge this attitude?"

What I like about Forster's questions is that they help establish continuity between ideologies that naturalize the rampant and extreme violence that litter the history of Guatemala and much of the everyday abuse that I witnessed in Sololá. Forster pushes us to consider why such abuse would look normal. She also asks us to think about the everyday practices of people who we might assume are "victims" (as well as "perpetrators") that would reinforce (or in some cases rebel against) the normality of violence. These questions helped orient me to be attentive to marks of violence in Santa Cruz.

One afternoon when I joined the stream of day laborers walking home on the paths in Santa Cruz, I heard two people fighting. As I neared the voices I noticed that no one was taking the normal path home, but that everyone was detouring to walk a longer way to the village. I asked one of the men passing me why everyone was going on the right path instead of the left, and he smiled sheepishly and shrugged, eager to escape my questions. I decided to take the right path also, and as I walked a little further, I came to a spot where I was able to see the steep path that everyone normally took, exposed on the side of the mountain. On it I saw a man and woman fighting. The woman was crying. The man was drunk. He was hitting her and trying to push her off the path. She was sitting down and sometimes moving out of his reach, but wailing and screaming at him the entire time. After watching a few minutes and seeing that everyone else was completely ignoring the incident, I too moved on. When I asked the next day someone told me that this woman had gone down to the dock to find her husband because word had reached her that he was very drunk and was unable to walk. He became infuriated that she would come and fetch him because he was a man and should be allowed to do what he wanted without having his wife interfere. What I saw on the mountain was the fight that ensued. Not to be considered an isolated incident, the day's gossip could contain stories about women running into the streets in the middle of the night crying and screaming that their husbands beat them.

Yet men were not the only perpetrators of violence. Gossip about abuse also frequently involved women attacking men. During my first few months in the field a teenager came to the health post, where my husband and I shared a workspace. The nurse was on vacation but he needed his wounds cleaned. Half of his face and one eye was swollen shut. Coagulating blood was caked into his hair. He had raw wounds in several places on his body. Apparently, he had come home drunk, and his mother, who objected to him drinking, beat him with a log from the fire to remind him never to drink again. The teachers in the school discovered that another child had been lashed with a cord by her mother.

Just as the violence of the civil war arguably naturalizes the macabre murders of women, these stories from everyday village life speak to how the hierarchy inherent to the social structure naturalizes family violence. Husbands beat wives. Wives react aggressively to their husbands. Both can beat their children. I never had the impression that anyone was in favor of family violence—not even those who were implicated as abusers. Nevertheless, the following story of a murdered mayoral candidate stands as a good illustration of what can happen to someone who tries to step in and interfere in another's family affairs, whether or not that meddling occurs during the pursuit of justice.

Just eight months before I arrived for my first field season a man who was running for mayor of Santa Cruz was murdered. Walking home from one of the aldeas after a campaign meeting, he apparently crossed paths with a drunken man who bore a grudge against him. The drunken man blamed the mayoral candidate, who was also a pastor, for translating at a court hearing between himself and his estranged wife. The drunken man apparently had abandoned his wife, and she, quite unusually, decided to sue him for his land as child and spousal support. When she won her case the drunken man considered that the mayoral candidate had a direct hand in stealing his property—namely, his wife and his land.

The mayoral candidate and the man got into a fight, and the man eventually ended up driving a piece of rebar through the mayoral candidate, essentially staking him to the spot. The attacker was either not alone or near home, but somehow a female person then boiled a huge caldron of water, which the man took and poured all over the mayoral candidate, apparently while he was still alive. After the mayoral candidate died they pushed him over a steep part of the path down into the bushes. The murderer apparently then went to a cantina and told people what he had done. Though the victim's family tried to press charges the murderer fled into the bush and hid until the police stopped looking for him. When the perpetrator was eventually brought into court he refused to admit what he had done and no one who had heard him confess or had helped him boil the water was willing to testify against him. He got off without serving any prison time. When I talked to the victim's sons about their father's death, they told me that they thought going through the official channels was the right thing to do, and what their father, who valued progress and education, would have wanted. They, therefore, did not seek revenge.

The crisis of justice is amplified by the fact that how to seek justice in most day-to-day situations in Guatemala seems to be particularly murky. In one instance that I watched unfold in Santa Cruz, a young man, Fernando, killed a romantic rival, who I will call Roberto. Fernando had been dating Bartola but she broke up with him. It now seemed that Roberto was interested in her, creating a situation of enmity between the two young men. One night, they both were drinking at a local tienda when Fernando claimed that Roberto either said something suggestive to him or looked at him in an antagonistic way. When Fernando was leaving for the night he walked by Roberto and pushed him. Roberto was not only drunk at that point, but was sitting on a wall. He fell about six feet backward off the wall and could not get up. The next day his family said that he was getting worse. The day after that they took him to the hospital, where he died. Fernando apologized to the family, claiming that he had not intentionally meant to kill Roberto, only to push him. The family pressed charges and said that they would have him arrested for murder unless Fernando made reparations. In this case he paid the family 40,000 Q, a little over three and half years of his full salary as a caretaker, to drop the charges.

Despite the fact that the two families agreed on how to settle the case, the arrangement left many in the village uneasy. Fernando had a very rich uncle, a land speculator, who gave him the cash he needed. People worried that now any member of the uncle's family could kill someone with impunity since they had the money to buy themselves out of the legal consequences. Others who were more sympathetic to the family emphasized that it would be a waste for Fernando to go jail, as it would ruin his own life without improving the situation for Roberto's family. Fernando didn't mean to kill

Roberto, and going to jail would not bring Roberto back. When I returned a year later, the incident was no longer talked about.

In fact, the changing of money followed any legal infraction far more frequently than judicial proceedings. When I was doing fieldwork in the hospital the police arrived on the tail of a major traffic accident. A young man had borrowed a pick-up truck from another family member, and loaded up two of his children, his mother-in-law, and his sister-in-law. On the highway he tried to pass a bus on a blind curve and had a head-on collision with a large truck. The truck suffered only minor damage, but the pick-up was destroyed. Everyone in it was taken to the ER. The mother-in-law was critical and one of the children died shortly after arrival. The driver broke both clavicles and was put into a cast that immobilized his upper body, but he survived, as did another of the children. When I arrived seven relatives and one policeman were in the ER. When the sister-in-law needed CPR, the family and policeman were all ushered out. After she died the family returned, but their focus shifted to trying to get her body back without it undergoing the obligatory autopsy. When the confusion subsided the main doctor on duty walked over to a woman who was talking to the driver. The doctor asked her if the driver was her husband and she said yes. Then he asked if she realized that her husband was going to jail. Did they tell you that, he asked? She looked bewildered and dumbfounded. The best thing to do is to work it out somehow, he told her. He said that he would file the papers to keep the driver in the hospital for twenty-four hours so that the police didn't arrest him that day. He would do her that favor but she needed to start trying to solve the problem now. The wife thanked him and left. I talked to the doctor after the emergency was over. He said that he noticed that the family, who were predominantly monolingual K'iche' speakers, were actively ignoring the policeman instead of trying to negotiate with him. They were going to have to pay to keep the husband out of jail, and he felt he needed to explain the process to them.

How the police were driven by money became even more apparent the longer I was in the hospital. In one particularly notable incident a man in a car turned into a gas station and hit a stationary motorcyclist who was waiting to pull out. The car driver loaded the motorcyclist into his car and brought him directly to the ER. He had a cell phone and allowed the motorcyclist, who arrived with a bone sticking out of his thigh, to call a family member. Within twenty-five minutes the family member and a lawyer had arrived at the ER. In the intervening time a policeman had also arrived on the scene and tried to get the preliminary details of the case. The driver of the car complained vociferously. Couldn't the policeman see that the motorcyclist was in pain? By being the motorcyclist's champion, the car driver delayed the paper from being filled out and, thereby, the case from becoming official. When the family member and lawyer arrived the driver continued his role as patient advocate, stressing his utmost concern for the motorcyclist and continuing to intervene on the motorcyclist's behalf. The family member talked to the motorcyclist and the lawyer talked to the policeman. They sought out the opinion of one doctor. The car driver then pointed out that it would take a long time to treat the motorcyclist and invited the family member and lawyer to come and have a soda pop with him. Much to the chagrin of the policeman they left together. After the drink the lawyer told the policeman that they would not be pressing charges against the car driver. Both the lawyer and the policeman then left. The car driver again went over and consoled his new best friend, the motorcyclist, promised to visit him while he was in the hospital, and left him alone with his relative.

When I asked one of the doctors about the interaction, he tried to explain what he considered to be its subtleties. The driver wanted to pay off the family directly, since it would be cheaper for him and easier than paying off the police. For this reason he was interested in appearing amiable, trustworthy, and concerned for the patient. Nevertheless, if the family asked for too much money, he could always threaten to walk. The family, for its part, wanted to make sure that they got as much money as possible out of the driver. They brought the lawyer to show that they were serious, and that if the driver did not pay they would press charges. Nevertheless, they did not want to press charges, because if they did the driver would end up paying off the police, not them, and they would end up both with an injured relative and poorer for having to pay the lawyer. The policeman, of course, wanted the family to press charges. Nevertheless, he was not able to forcibly introduce himself into the situation, especially because of the presence of the lawyer. When the driver invited the lawyer and the relative for a pop, there was nothing the policeman could do but wait and see if the bargain was struck.

Indeed, I would go so far as to say that both the police and the law in Guatemala created as much or more injustice than they solved. One of the popular moral tales I heard repeated in Santa Cruz highlighted the tension between doing the right thing and the way the legal system worked. Luis, a teenage boat driver, was taking a group of passengers from Santa Cruz to Panajachel. The boat dock in Pana abutted a public swimming beach that was popular with visitors to the town. Many visitors unfortunately did not realize that boat drivers cannot see swimmers in the water. Because of this hazard the rule is that each driver should have a lookout in the front of the boat. On the day that Luis broke this rule he was following another boat arriving from another town. Everyone in his boat saw a tourist swimming, and then saw the boat in front of them run the tourist over. They called to Luis, who slowed down and circled back to find the swimmer. The passengers spotted him and pulled him into the boat. He had been sliced across the back, was losing blood, and was not in good shape. They got the tourist to the hospital, where he was stabilized, transported, and survived. Luis, however, was arrested and held in jail. His father communicated with the boat driver who had hit the swimmer but that man refused to admit his guilt. No one in either boat was willing to get involved in the case, as they didn't want to make enemies of either boat driver. In the end Luis's father borrowed a lot of money and paid off the tourist's family, who was from Guatemala City. They dropped the charges and Luis came home.

The lesson learned from this incident was so obvious that later when a tourist was hit in Santa Cruz by a boat driver who had no idea anyone was in the water, those watching from the shore were reluctant to do anything. What if the man died? Would they be arrested? Indeed, right before I left, a man drowned in just a few feet of water on a docked boat because a load of corrugated aluminum shifted and trapped him on the bow of the boat, which then sunk under the weight. Despite the fact that there were several adults on the shore, no one got in the water to try to free him. He drowned in front of one of his children.

Fleeing the scene or not getting involved are by no means marginalized experiences. Victims of hit-and-run accidents were upsettingly commonplace in the ER. Abandoning someone in the street seemed especially egregious since getting help in a timely manner might help the injured survive. When I asked one of the doctors in the ER why there were so many hit-and-runs, he blamed it on the police. He said that most of the hit-and-runs that they received were cases where a man got drunk and then laid down in the road to sleep it off. As driving conditions are not optimal in the country the driver probably was unable to see the man in the road and hit him. In Guatemala the category of manslaughter does not exist, and someone who runs over a drunk sleeping in the road in the middle of the night receives the same sentence as someone who takes a machete and intentionally hacks apart his neighbor. And even if the drunk were not to die, as soon as you get to the hospital the police will arrest you. You have to have lots of resources available to bribe them or you will never get out. As the doctor rationalized it the moment you hit someone, you have to choose between spending the rest of your life in jail, condemning your family to live without support, or to drive away. For him, it came down to a choice between a drunken person you do not know and your own families. Who would choose the stranger? In a rather candid moment he told me that if I was not prepared to drive away from an accident, then I should not drive in Guatemala.[17]

Guatemala may have a system of laws on the books, but it is difficult to argue that those laws constitute any reasonable form of protection for the populace—particularly against violence. Similar to those living in the Brazilian _favelas_ that Donna Goldstein (2003:196) describes, "populations … are willing to accept any justice, as long as it is directed at the right person." In the absence of any coherent judicial system, people take matters into their own hands, and violence is undoubtedly one of the main tools that is used to bring justice. Lynching of state representatives in areas outside of the capitol has been documented since colonial times (McCreery 1994) and the threat to lynch was a pervasive tool that the populace used to mediate their relations with local State representatives. Toward the end of my first year of fieldwork, people began to revolt against the mayor of San Pablo.[18] Though I heard many different stories, they all conjoined in that the mayoral administration was suffering from an untenable amount of corruption. Apparently, when the mayor was running for office he was approached by a man, whom we will call Guillermo. Guillermo asked to be appointed secretary for the municipality in the mayor's new administration. Guillermo was not from San Pablo and had been kicked out of a prior administration in his natal village for being corrupt. True to form, Guillermo offered to pay the mayor a large sum of money if he was given the job of secretary. The mayor acceded. Two years into the administration the mayor apparently had built a new house and bought a new pick-up truck, the mayor's brother was building a new house, and Guillermo had bought up all of the waterfront property in the village that he could get his hands on. The story began to go south when Guillermo commanded that the water for the village be shut off. As the village sits atop a hill, and there is no sewer system, all of the water used in the village eventually drains off into and erodes the lakefront property that Guillermo had purchased. Cutting off the water was his recourse to save his land. Living without running water was an incredible hardship (let alone a health nightmare) and the people marched angrily on the municipality. They demanded that both the mayor and the secretary resign and, in an absence of a resignation, threatened to kill them. The mayor, however, refused to resign and called in national authorities. When I left, MINUGUA was holding citizenry workshops in the locale. Their perspective was that, despite the fact that the mayor might be corrupt, lynching was not part of the mechanics of democracy. They alleged that over time, running the mayor out of office would only weaken the democratic process, as an elected official could only be rightfully removed through judicial processes. The State had agreed to prosecute some of the embezzlement. But two years later when I again left the field, the mayor had weathered the crisis, new elections were coming up, and the State had yet to charge him with any crime.

This incident in San Pablo reflects well the tensions between democracy and justice. On the one hand, MINUGUA articulates well that you cannot only apply due process when it is convenient for you. If one wants a democratic and fair society, then one has to follow the rules all of the time. On the other hand, it is glaringly obvious that no bureaucratic official should be able to summarily cut off the water supply to the village because it is convenient to him. And it is inhumane to expect villagers to live without water while the bureaucracy attempts to figure out how to turn the water back on through legitimate means.[19] This incident also illustrates well the strict division between indigenous villages and the institution of government. Regardless of ethnicity, or the fact that local mayors are elected, little progress seems to have been made to transform government into an institution that represents, rather than oppresses, people.

But threats of lynching are also used to galvanize political positions. My work at the health post in San Marcos during my second year was upset by lynching threats against the nurse, who was a Tz'utujil man from a nearby village. The circumstances surrounding the case are murky, but the problem essentially grew out of the distribution of free food donated by World Vision, a private voluntary organization, to the families of malnourished children. World Vision had formed a committee to locally administer its donations. The nurse at the health post, however, was in charge of deciding precisely which children were malnourished, supposedly by comparing the children's height and weight to the developmental chart. Then one day, the director of the Ministry of Health office in Sololá received a letter from some citizens in San Marcos saying that the nurse was somehow abusing the system of food dispersal and that if the Ministry of Health did not remove him from his post immediately, the citizens of San Marcos would mob the health post and lynch the nurse.

I heard several interpretations of what precisely caused the problem. One person told me that the nurse decided to distribute the food equitably among all families with children, because it seemed obscene that some families received one hundred pounds of corn and some families received none. The nurse thought that equitable distribution was a fairer system and would prevent both jealousy and wasted food. Another person told me that the nurse was trying to link food distribution to vaccination coverage. One of the primary pressures on the nurses in the health posts is to make sure that every baby gets vaccinated, and the evaluation of their own performance is closely linked to the vaccination coverage they achieve. In a country where many parents refuse vaccination, this is a difficult task and, not unreasonably, nurses might create incentives to get the population to comply. The nurse himself claimed that the advisory council to distribute the food had been hijacked by an individual who intended to run for mayor during the coming elections (one year later). He came to the nurse and proposed that they distribute the food to his supporters and use it to buy votes. Because the nurse refused to participate in the plan, the man launched a campaign to get rid of him. He knew that with the nurse out of the way he would have free reign to control the food for at least several months, perhaps enough time to buy his way into the mayoral office. The director, who received the letter, pulled the nurse from the site immediately. Though the nurse had over ten years of experience working in that village and several allies from San Marcos wrote contravening letters to the Ministry supporting him, the director felt that he could not risk the political turmoil that might ensue if he sent the nurse back.

The threat to lynch in this instance was unlike the others that I heard about or witnessed while I was in Guatemala, [20] because it lacked any "mob mentality." Instead, the vigilante edict arrived in a missive sent through the post. It is interesting to me that in the absence of the angry crowd the threat was still considered legitimate. Perhaps because the nurse was a state representative (i.e., a traditional "victim" of lynching), the director found it believable. Regardless of its legitimacy, invoking lynching as part of everyday diplomacy resulted in an absence of local healthcare from the village for almost six months. Anyone who needed medical attention was forced to walk or to pay extra money to travel to the next village to get attention.

Living in an environment where "anything is possible" made me hesitant to assume that even mundane activities were safe. People were not worried enough about the consequences of killing a neighbor, cutting off the entire village from water or from healthcare, embezzling funds, etc., to deter them from such transgressions. In all fairness, worrying about the consequences of crime was perhaps impractical, given that these consequences were so unpredictable. Perhaps what was most scary for me in this situation was that violence was not taboo—instead it seemed almost commonplace. So while I undoubtedly believe that the current spate of gruesome murders of women are connected to a heavily armed populace that was habitualized to committing violent acts over an extended period of civil war, it does seem important to note that violence—even gruesome violence—is not new in Guatemala.

Day-to-Day Life: Exploitation in Santa Cruz

Sitting on the crammed Friday market bus, piled high with food and people, I watched a man dressed in a suit, with gold cufflinks, gold teeth, and a Billy Graham combed-back hairdo, board the bus. He stood at the front and began his pitch. After greeting his audience and introducing himself he began to talk about people who you know. They get up at 5:30 or 6:00 AM and say that they can't eat so early because their stomach cannot handle the food. They start their day's work, and then around 10:00 AM they stop and have some tortillas for "breakfast." He marks this word as if it were absurd. Breakfast, as we all know, should be eaten when you get up, not at 10:00 AM. Of course when lunch time rolls around, they aren't hungry. They keep working until 2:00 or 3:00 PM, at which point they sit down and have more tortillas. Though this is supposed to be "lunch," the meal is eaten so late that they couldn't possibly eat again at 6:00 or 7:00 PM, so they end up skipping dinner. When they wake up the next morning their stomachs are off again and they don't want to eat. This habit, the salesman proclaimed, is the source of *gastritis*—it is the basis of constant stomach pain. He was selling a product that, mixed with a little bit of water, could relieve this pain and help you get back onto the road of health and good eating. Throughout his discourse he looked to the back of the bus and nodded at potential customers, who were clambering to get at the product. "Wait one minute and let me finish," he informed them. Turning around to look, I was never able to identify whom he had been talking to.

This man on the bus came to represent for me the confusion about food and hunger that was a constant theme during my fieldwork. Scheper-Hughes (1992) prepared me for the idea that hunger was not always represented as such, yet I went to the field with little idea of what hunger in Guatemala might look like. My notion of "malnourished" initially came to be formed by children I saw in the hospital with pellagra or by the nurses in the health district describing cases of acute childhood malnutrition. Yet, after living in Santa Cruz for over a year I realized that these cases were the extremes and that the real evidence of hunger was not as grotesque. Rather, the real threat was the much more subtle, but insidious toll that came from not having enough to eat everyday.

As we saw in the previous section the body is a sensitive indicator of ideologies concerning violence. The violent politics of Guatemala are equally as evident in the shortness that surrounded me in Santa Cruz as they are in the maimed bodies that kidnappers dump on the side of the road. According to the WHO Expert Report on Physical Status (1995), the better term for the low height-to-age stature that we find in Guatemala is "stunted." Stunting happens when children 5 and under fail to grow "as a result of suboptimal health and/or nutritional conditions" (116). This lack of growth is never made up for and, consequently, adult stature stands as a testament to poor childhood conditions. In a country like Guatemala the report tells us that the term "chronic malnutrition" is often substituted for stunting. The report also tells us that rates for stunting in the developing world among the 5-and-under crowd range from 5 to 65 percent. The most current statistics for Guatemala (taken in 2002) in the WHO Global Database on Child Growth and Malnutrition list an estimated 63.5 percent of children age 5 and under who live in the highlands are two standard deviations below the mean for height. Disturbingly, 34.3 percent are three or more standard deviations below the mean. The seriousness of the WHO data is supported all over the web. UNICEF reports that one out of every two children in Guatemala is chronically malnourished, and that number could be substantially higher for indigenous children (Nybo 2009). Lest we doubt that malnutrition is a problem across the lifespan, World Bank (2003) data show that malnutrition among children in Guatemala is closely correlated with poverty of a child's family.

Over time I began to see what the chronic shortage of food in people's lives actually looked like in the everyday. When Santa Cruz sponsored a soccer team from a beach town about three and a half hours away by bus, no food was available for the players once they got to Santa Cruz. Not only was lunch not part of the deal, but, literally, no one was selling anything for them to eat or to drink. If they wanted something they would have had to have walked to town or the dock from the soccer fields and all that was available there was soda and chips. A woman who traveled to classes in Antigua (about four hours away) every Saturday gave me a detailed description of what her life was like while studying outside of the village. Eating, however, was conspicuously absent from her narrative, so I asked her when she found time to eat. She said that she wasn't comfortable bringing lunch and eating it on the bus, and once she got to Antigua there was just no time to eat. She normally had a soda and chips to tide over her hunger until she got home again (sometimes eighteen to twenty-four hours later). I ran into an acquaintance that was walking back from visiting his grandmother, who lived one village over. Since he had left in the morning and had been gone all day, I assumed he must have had lunch with his grandmother. When I asked he told me that, on the contrary, his grandmother was poor and he hadn't eaten anything. I was surprised that a very elderly woman could go all day without food. He explained to me that his grandmother had periodically left him and gone into the kitchen to tend to the fire. He assumed that she was eating bites every time she did that.

Food in Santa Cruz was more expensive and less available than in other villages around the lake because Santa Cruz is relatively isolated. It was impossible to reach the village by car, so all external purchases had to be carried on someone's back down a mountain, or brought by boat across the lake and then carried up part of a mountain. Transport adds an extra cost onto most everything purchased in the village. It also creates a crucial barrier to affordability for poor villagers who could not afford frequent trips to the Sololá market to get cheap prices.[21] The costs for vendors to get to Santa Cruz also meant that there was no weekly market held in the village, limiting people's ability to buy fresh fruits and vegetables. For daily goods there were a number of small shops located throughout the village that sold basics such as soda and several varieties of chips, cookies, and gum. The larger ones had obtained refrigerators from the soda companies; the smaller ones offered drinks at room temperature. In a typical shop you might also find small cans of beans and juice, bouillon cubes, toilet paper, candles, and sugar. A larger store might stock margarine, instant coffee, bread rolls, beer, cigarettes, and matches. When I arrived in Santa Cruz two of the tiendas bought some fruits and vegetables in the Sololá market and resold them, but there was no constant supply. The produce that you could purchase in the village (primarily onions, tomatoes, and bananas) was not in good condition and was overpriced. When I last left, ambulatory vendors from another village had started selling house-to-house. One man from the village had started to sell some fruits and vegetables from a stall on the main square. The high school had also begun a project of purchasing fruits and vegetables at the market on Friday and reselling them throughout the week. Nevertheless, the quality of this produce was normally much worse than that in the market, seeing as it had been moved by bus, then boat, then carried on someone's back to its new venue, where it then suffered from a lack of refrigeration.[22] It also was significantly more costly than the same produce at the market. Sellers not only had to pay for the extra transport costs, but had to make some sort of profit to keep their businesses going. This means that people who most needed access to good fruits and vegetables—i.e., people who were too poor to go to the market and purchase them themselves—only had the opportunity to buy expensive produce that was frequently in bad shape.

The challenges of affording food in Santa Cruz are perhaps best illustrated by the example of corn. Corn is the main staple and is consumed as tortillas during every meal. Sometimes a meal might consist of only tortillas with a little salt or chili rubbed on them. Other meals might consist of tortillas with beans or eggs or soup. Many of the more wealthy families in town own land on which to produce their own corn. When no family member is available to clean the land and tend the corn, day laborers are hired to do the work.[23] The next best strategy to growing your own corn is to purchase it in bulk and store it. At the end of the season, the price of corn is about 40 percent more than after harvest. Families that cannot afford to buy corn in bulk and have no land (i.e., the poorest families) must purchase it locally from one of the many tiendas, and frequently must pay double the bulk price.

The exceedingly poor water quality in Santa Cruz only exacerbated the problems with food. Unlike some of the surrounding villages, municipal water storage tanks were located within, instead of above or outside, the village. Since there was no sewer or waste disposal system, sewage could seep not only into the pipes, but into the tanks themselves. During my second year of fieldwork water quality in Santa Cruz was the poorest in the entire health district and the Ministry of Health had filed a court case against the mayor, whose responsibility it was to clean it up. Though the Ministry was willing to send a technician to teach the workers at the municipality how to install a chlorinator and purify the water, the mayor was unwilling to do anything about the situation. The generally problematic water supply meant that most adults and children suffered from some sort of intestinal parasite or infection, which prevented them from taking full nutritional advantage of the scant food that they were eating.

Key to understanding the poverty that made buying what little food was available difficult were the constant relations of exploitation that governed villagers' lives. While in a few instances individual Cruceños were in a position to be exploiters, in general they came out on the short end of the stick. At first this was difficult for me to understand, because in some ways Cruceños are in a much better position to make a living than sister villagers in their district. The influx of gringos to the area has transformed the economy and meant that two generations of men and women have been exempt from migrating to the plantations for seasonal work.[24] During the late 1970s and early 1980s, villagers in Santa Cruz began to sell lakefront land to wealthy Guatemalans from the city, who built vacation homes, known locally as "chalets." The first chalet built in Santa Cruz included a grassy front yard equipped with a helicopter pad so that the owner and his family could quickly travel from the city to their vacation home, unencumbered by the fact that at the time, canoe was a popular means of reaching Santa Cruz. As of 2003 there were almost fifty chalets in Santa Cruz, twelve of which were the permanent residence of their owners and another ten of which were occupied at least six months of the year. Santa Cruz also saw its own popularity as a tourist destination grow and four foreign-owned hotels were operating during my fieldwork.

The development of local land fueled a construction boom, and the majority of the chalets in Santa Cruz have been built by local laborers (men).[25] Each chalet also needs to have a *guardian*, a man who is responsible for protecting the property, especially when the owners are not there.[26] One of the advantages of being a guardian is that it is full-time, stable employment with "benefits,"[27] and the majority of guardianes work unsupervised for several, if not most, months of the year. In addition to benefits most guardianes earn more than day laborers—temporary workers employed in activities as diverse as building roads, grounds work at the chalets, and agricultural work. One gringo land owner in Santa Cruz has designed such an extensive garden system, that he is the main employer in the town, and on any one day employs between twenty and one hundred men.

This transformation both benefitted and challenged villagers. Having sources of cash labor available in the village relieved many of the burdens associated with migration. Families no longer needed to be separated, income could be earned throughout the year, no upfront capital was needed to get a job, the disease burden of working in the village was much lower than in many of the plantations, children's studies were not disrupted, and the dangers of travel and being among strangers were allayed. Despite the influx of possibility, pay for "unskilled" labor was still poor. The going rate for day labor was about $3.20 US, and the guardianes earned between $4.40 and $6.40 US a day. Even in a place like Santa Cruz where cost of living was generally low, these salaries were not particularly generous.[28] The arrival of foreigners did open up wage-labor opportunities for women, as discussed in chapter 1. But the arrival of foreigners has also alienated Cruceños from one resource they had depended on for millennia: land. Land near the lakeshore is the flattest land available in Santa Cruz and, logically, the best for agriculture. Families, however, sold off that land and moved their cultivation to the steep hillsides, which not only increased erosion, but meant decreased yield for the families.[29] Selling off agricultural land has also impacted the traditional inheritance system, where both males and females received land from their parents. Yet many people were bedazzled by what they considered to be the fortunes that they were being offered for their family land. Many intended to (and some did) sell and then buy other pieces of land farther from the shore with the money they received. Others thought that the amounts they were getting for their land was so generous that they would be able to give their children inheritance of equal value in cash. Considering inflation in Guatemala, this was not an accurate perception. Many families were now struggling to put together any inheritance at all. Land relations in Guatemala have never been uncontentious,[30] but many are upset at how out of reach buying land has become for them. Sellers now charge premium prices for plots that foreigners would never want, knowing that their neighbors can raise the money by selling some of their inheritance. Prices have gone up for almost any resource that foreigners use, since everyone knows that selling high might be an option.

Another detail to add to the pot is that economic opportunities for Cruceños were also frequently more constrained than they were for others around the lake. Probably due to its geographic isolation, Cruceños frequently lacked the connections that they would need to be more economically viable. For example, Santa Cruz serves as a plantation of sorts for wealthy indigenous people in San Pedro and Santiago. Buyers from these Tz'utujil towns located across the lake have access to processors and markets that Cruceños lack. In 2002, when coffee prices were so bad that many families refused to pick, a Pedrano showed up in a private boat with a group of men. He walked around town finding people who owned coffee plots, purchased the yearly rights to those plots very cheaply, and sent his men over to pick the coffee right then and there. With their bundle in hand they returned to San Pedro to process it. In another example that year, a few men from Santiago showed up and bought as many harvests from the avocado trees as Cruceños were willing to sell. Remarkably, they bought the avocados formed, but still green. They got them at a very inexpensive price because they argued to the Cruceños that not all avocados would mature, would be free of worms, or would be left by the birds. Many people thought it was better to sell today cheaply than to wait until tomorrow when a substantial portion of their crop might be ruined. The men from Santiago said that they needed the avocados because some buyer was making and marketing a new conditioner. As these stories demonstrate Santa Cruz has become a site for the extraction of raw materials—in many cases Cruceños are even denied the right to charge for their labor. If there is any profit to be made in coffee or avocados, the indigenous middle men who know where and when to contact the growers are reaping the benefits. In Santa Cruz most people are beholden to the few buyers who come to the village, and there is little room for Cruceños to negotiate a good selling price.

Lack of connections also kept Cruceños from working in *maquilas* (factories) (Goldin 2001) or migrating to the US, both normative activities in many parts of Guatemala.[31] Cruceños told me that in order to make a profit from a maquila job, you need a relative or friend who works or lives near the factory. Without that you have no one to stay with until your job comes through, and even if you were to get a job it would be difficult to make any profit without a cheap place to live and easy transport. Similarly, Cruceños lacked friends and relatives to live with in the US. But perhaps the greatest barrier to migrating to the US was that Santa Cruz lacked a *coyote*, the individual whose job it is to get workers across the border. People told me that a few years ago, a man showed up claiming to be a coyote. He held a general meeting and said that he could take a limited number of men to the US and would give priority to those who paid first. Several families scraped together the money to send someone. The coyote took the money, told the men to be ready to travel on an assigned day, when he would return to pick them up. Of course, he never reappeared. Even if one is not defrauded upfront, stories abound of men being taken across the border to Mexico, driven out into the desert, and then robbed and shot by the coyote. The men are never heard from again, and the coyote returns claiming they arrived safely and looking for his next group of victims.[32]

Santa Cruz's lack of connections has figured prominently into its poverty by making most Cruceños hopelessly dependent on middle men who can exploit them. On the most literal level the fact that it was the only major village in Sololá not accessible by car meant that most villagers were dependent on buying from the few families that could afford to transport goods. Even items like soft drinks, which come with the price already printed on the front, were re-priced by store owners. Basic staples sometimes cost twice as much as at nearby markets. The lack of connections also meant Cruceños were exploited by middle men from other villages looking for cheap agricultural goods. These middle men had access to buyers and markets that were unknown to those in Santa Cruz. While transformations in the economy that accompanied the influx of foreigners meant that one no longer had to migrate to obtain a cash income, the salaries paid to workers nationwide are by no means sufficient to overcome poverty.

In sum, people in Santa Cruz faced real everyday challenges concerning poverty and availability of food. Nevertheless, it is still remarkable to me that that people were slowly starving to death without ever talking about it. Never did I hear anyone protest about lack of food; I never even heard a conversation about chronic hunger.[33] When hunger was referenced it was disguised, as illustrated by the entrepreneur's pitch that started this section. The schedule of meals where you only eat twice a day is codified as a preference instead of a result of poverty. In addition, the pain that you feel in your stomach is medically pathologized. Your problem, this sales man would tell you, is not that you don't have food. Your problem is that you reject good food because you are sick.

This tension between hunger and sickness again brings us back to Scheper-Hughes, who points out that the social implications of the

two are decidedly different: "A hungry body needs food. A sick ...
body needs medications. A hungry body exists as a potent critique of
the society in which it exists. A sick body implicates no one. Such is
the special privilege of sickness as a *neutral* social role, its exemptive
status. In sickness there is (ideally) no blame, no guilt, no responsibility. Sickness falls into the moral category of bad things that 'just
happen' to people" (1992:174). In her analysis, sickness is neutral
in that it provides no critique of the State or the structural violence
(Farmer 1992, 2003) that characterizes a society riddled by such inequality that certain members are forced to slowly starve to death,
day by day. Hunger, on the other hand, implies injustice. She goes
further to argue that the poor in Brazil willingly collude in making hunger neutral by medicalizing it themselves. The poor, as also
demonstrated here, view their hunger as a sickness—be it *nervos* in
Brazil or gastritis in Guatemala.

Why would villagers in Santa Cruz "come not only to acquiesce,
but even to participate in their own undoing," as Scheper-Hughes
(1992:172) puts it? Why would someone slowly starving to death,
or watching their family starving to death, not scream, yell, protest, or at least dramatically and publically faint from hunger pains
as peasants in Brazil did during the 1960s? Scheper-Hughes argues
that "relations of power" are masked such that the poor do not
clearly understand "their situation in the world," and that middle-
class ideologies (such as the trust in biomedicine in this case), are
co-opted by all classes (171). While a class-based analysis resonates
with many aspects of the situation in Guatemala, it mutes the enormous role of violence in making starvation appear ordinary.[34]

The fear that everyday violence generates has made the world
beyond Santa Cruz less accessible and normalized a situation where
there is, at least during some point in the year, a lack of food. While
violence certainly can come to your doorstep, the extensiveness of
violence in Guatemala created a situation where leaving one's home
and village was not only difficult or expensive, it was often dangerous. So fear keeps one close to home when possible, but also stops
one from getting involved with unknown people. Eric Wolf's (1957)
discussion of the inaccessibility of Mayan "closed-corporate peasant
communit[ies]" underscores how closing the community to outsiders was a security strategy crafted in response to an abusive state apparatus. The danger for a villager going afoot was highlighted for me
when I asked one Cruceño why he didn't wear *traje* (native clothing) anymore. He told me that he might consider wearing it in the
village, but now he could go to town (Sololá or Panajachel) without

anyone knowing who he was. Before, whenever he left the village, the design of his pants and shirt told everyone that he was not from that town. He considered safety to be found in anonymity and not drawing attention to himself.

Shortages of food year after year have made "short but healthy" (Bogin and Loucky 1997), an idea now rejected by those who study malnutrition and growth, appear not only possible, but common. And how could it be otherwise? There was no visual evidence like that which Lynn Meisch (1995) describes among indigenous in highland Ecuador, where younger generations tower over their elders. Indeed, it would be difficult to posit that stunting had ever been less any time in the last five hundred years, because growing taller would only be possible if several generations of indigenous poor had been able to count on relative abundance. And in Santa Cruz there was no evidence of anyone socialized to think short and hungry is remarkable.

We can now return to the man who boarded the bus to tell us that we might be suffering from gastritis. As I pointed out above the palpable lack of food experienced by most poor indigenous people in Sololá is not at all unusual—rather, it is the norm. It is counterintuitive to look to the normal to explain something that seems aberrant (i.e., pain in your stomach and a rejection of food). Sickness, however, is something aberrant. For many of the poor, indigenous villagers who make use of the public bus, sickness could make sense of their trouble, where hunger could not.

Violence, Uncertainty, and Birth Choice

What does a broken justice system and a fear of what might be waiting for you around every corner have to do with seeking obstetric care? And if people are so poor, why aren't they jumping at the chance to give birth in a hospital that provides free obstetric care, and staff who have undergone recent and extensive training? Charles Briggs (2004) argues that gossip and conspiratorial theories that often sweep through the lives of the poor reflect the fact that almost unimaginable violence and injustice are possible in their lives. In this chapter I have tried to show what some of that unimaginable violence and injustice has looked like. Behaviors like not seeking out or trusting a skilled attendant in a government-sponsored hospital have to be understood within this context where the unimaginable is often fused with reality.

As we have seen, the body is a sensitive indicator of ideologies concerning violence in Guatemala. The particularly gruesome murders of women that continue to take place to this day help us understand how the legacy of violence has inured perpetrators to the full humanity of women. The burned bodies that show up in villages around the country represent the comingling between perpetrator and victim—methods so recently used against villagers have been embraced as their own weapons to defend themselves. The violent politics of Guatemala are as easily seen in the stature of its indigenous population as they are on the front pages of the tabloids that report the growing toll of murder.

The vulnerable position of the body in both taking on and representing the violence in Guatemala makes the intervention to reduce maternal mortality particularly problematic. Women giving birth need to be safe—indeed, the consequences of letting a woman's body be harmed during this process could be particularly egregious. So for a family that attends a birth, handing over a woman in the throes of labor to hospital personnel would be exceptionally difficult. Given the palpable context of violence that makes even the unthinkable plausible, we can now understand why villagers are reasonably reluctant to fully embrace a policy that results in them ceding any tiny bit of control over their bodies that they maintain.

Chapter 6

PRAYING FOR A GOOD OUTCOME
STAYING AT HOME DURING OBSTETRIC PROBLEMS

The part of my research that seemed so counterintuitive and so compelling was this simple question: Why would a woman die at home rather than seek help for a birthing problem? Were the Kaqchikel people in Santa Cruz a group of ideological radicals who felt, as one observer often put it, "tradition is thicker than blood"? Would they really rather die than break their traditions?

Several of the alternative lay theories that I heard bantered among health workers were no more palatable. Was the Kaqchikel village structure so patriarchal that women had no choice and were just subjugated to the whims of their husbands and fathers-in-law? Were women's lives so expendable that it was easier to let a woman die and replace her with another woman than to save her? Surely there were some bad relationships between couples and women and their in-laws, but "bad relationships" didn't come close to elucidating the reasons for the maternal deaths that I witnessed. Nor did it seem that the men involved in these scenarios were untouched when women died. The hypothesis that life means nothing in Guatemala and that one more or one less death is really irrelevant also fell short. Compared to almost any privileged background, death in a Mayan village is commonplace, but it does not follow that people are automatically inured to it. Years of oppression and civil war have not succeeded in erasing the importance of immediate kin ties or the meaning of life.

While it made sense that women preferred the system of home-birth in a familiar setting to giving birth alone, on their backs, in a rather public place, this did not address why women did not go to the hospital as soon as they encountered a problem. Why wouldn't a woman suffering during a birth that is obviously outside the bounds of "normal" immediately seek care in the hospital? Why would she wait?

My first tack to try to understand why women "prefer" to die at home failed miserably. During interviews with women in the villages I asked several iterations of the same question: "If a woman dies from a pregnancy-related complication, is it better that she die at home or in the hospital?" I was almost certain that people would unequivocally answer "at home." During my conversations with health workers they told me that people were too attached to their own traditions to use the hospital. The literature I read also advised me that cost might be a determining factor in hospital use, because it costs money to get to the hospital, even if treatment was free. Wouldn't people reason that it might be too costly to go to the hospital and, therefore, prefer to wait and see if they get better at home? I myself had seen the resistance to the autopsy after Rosario had died, and I fully expected some people to think that dying at home was much nicer because at least no ugly body cutting (i.e., an autopsy) would follow the death.

In the end, however, this question turned out to be useless because women did not want to answer it.[1] The small amount of responses I did receive revealed how nonsensical the question was. What was important to the women was whether or not you died, not where you died. As many pointed out, it is just the same to die in your house as it is in the hospital, because the end result is that you are dead. When I pushed the point of the cost of dying in the hospital versus the cost of dying at home, everyone admitted that it cost more to die in the hospital. One woman who had answered that it was the same to die in both places retorted that the question I asked was about where it is better to die, not where it costs more to die. For her the only question worth answering was do you want to die or not? Once you are dead it doesn't matter where you are.

Where was the resistance to the hospital coming from, then? My next strategy was to try to use the ubiquitous saying "the hospital is the place that you go to die" as a probe. But talking to people about that saying did little to help me understand who was willing or unwilling to go to the hospital. In fact, a double discourse existed: the same woman would tell me that the hospital is the place that you go to die and that she herself would go if she thought that she was dying. Woman told me that they trust that the doctor is a professional who knows his/her work, yet responded with uncertainty as to how confident they were that a birthing problem could be solved at the hospital. Nevertheless, the women whom I interviewed did not see a choice; regardless of whether they thought that they would survive, they said that they would have to go to the hospital anyway. The conclusion I drew from these conversations was that the hospital was considered a last resort.

Abandoning the idea that women do not seek emergency care because they prefer to die at home or because they refuse to use the hospital, this chapter goes on to explore some social factors that influence a woman to remain at home when she experiences a life-threatening pregnancy-related problem. The foundation of the birthing process is the relationship between a woman and her family and the midwife who attends the birth. I have artificially divided my discussion into factors that influence midwives' interpretations and responses to birthing "problems" and factors that impact women and their families' desires to run off to the hospital for help. In reality, these factors are mutually constitutive and there is a feedback loop between the midwife, who knows that her client family does not want to go to the hospital unless absolutely necessary, and the client family, who does not want to go to the hospital and trusts that the midwife will be able to use her skills and powers to make the birth come out right.

Why Midwives Do Not Make Referrals

Over the two years that I worked in Sololá, iyoma were required to attend monthly training meetings with someone who staffed the Ministry of Health posts or centers.[2] These monthly meetings followed a national curriculum to teach iyoma to identify an obstetric problem early enough to make a timely referral. They also introduced iyoma to new policies, such as the importance of making emergency plans for individual birthing women and organizing the community to prepare for an emergency evacuation.[3]

No one within the Safe Motherhood campaign ever told me that they thought these classes were really altering midwifery practices. The iyoma would learn in class that if the placenta did not come out within thirty minutes of the child being born, then you must transport. Nevertheless, women arrived at the hospital with placentas that had been retained for five or six hours, or they died at home after the placenta remained in their womb all night. Other women had arrived with one arm emerging from the birth canal, with what the midwives knew long before was a transverse birth. The problem that health workers had trouble reconciling is that none of those conditions were emergent: rather they took hours to unfold. In each of these cases, health workers concluded, iyoma waited well beyond what they were taught is the danger sign before referring their clients.

Safe Motherhood in general has been at a loss to understand why all of the work with midwives has failed to change practices.[4] Can midwives just not understand what they are being taught? The imagined intransigence of midwives' practices does not, in my mind, reflect on midwives' knowledge or lack of it. Rather, it speaks to the fact that the global organizations, NGOs, and ministries of health involved in Safe Motherhood do not have the authority that they imagine. Anthropologists have documented in a variety of settings the propensity of biomedical providers to assume that their knowledge is better than or dominant over "traditional" knowledge.[5] Yet in many instances, this is just not the case. Looking at why iyoma in Sololá tended to disregard the information they were taught about when to refer can help us understand this.

Midwives as Empirical Learners

One of the fundamental reasons why iyoma did not embrace the guidelines promoted by the Safe Motherhood campaign is that the guidelines frequently did not seem to be true. The Safe Motherhood campaign was heavily reliant on international research to establish its policies. This created a disjuncture between theory and the everyday practice in Sololá. This disjuncture was fatal for the Safe Motherhood campaign, because iyoma, like many other midwives, base their own understandings of pregnancy and birth on experiences at the local level. The disjuncture both meant that information appeared to be incorrect and that many of the campaign's spoken or written policies were contradicted in practice. These contradictions, in turn, undermined iyoma's trust in the information that the Safe Motherhood campaign was disseminating. The example of how to treat post-caesarean deliveries provides an excellent example of this tension

One of the guidelines promoted by the Safe Motherhood campaign that was particularly contentious among iyoma, their clients, and their families was the mandate that all women who have a scar from a c-section need to deliver subsequent pregnancies in the hospital. The Safe Motherhood campaign based this recommendation on the fact that literature has shown that post-caesarean pregnancies involved the potential risk of the scar ripping open (i.e., uterine rupture) (Justus Hofmeyr, Say, and Metin Gulmezoglu 2005). The Ministry of Health distributed graphic materials that showed c-section scars as a sign of danger necessitating automatic referral to the hospital (MSPAS et al. 1996).

When I asked iyoma informally if a woman who had a previous c-section should only deliver in the hospital, their responses repeatedly consisted of a list of names of women who had delivered by caesarean, and then had subsequent vaginal births at home without any problem at all. Iyoma pointed out that their own experiences delivering post-caesarean pregnancies contradicted the information that they were receiving from health workers, who told them that post-caesarean deliveries were dangerous. If they were so dangerous, why didn't women have a problem delivering? The obvious implication was that the information in the Safe Motherhood campaign just wasn't true.

If we look at the numbers we can see how small the probability actually is that an *iyom* in this area will ever witness a uterine rupture. Of all of the villages that I worked in, San Marcos had the best quality data on birthing in the village; an average of sixty-four babies were born each year and seven iyoma were actively attending. Records for obstetric operations in the Sololá hospital existed for four years, and during those years, a total of ten women from San Marcos received c-sections. So an iyom may deliver at the most a few women per year who have c-section scars, but quite likely may not even have one post-caesarean delivery per year. Keep this in mind when we look at the likelihood that a scar will burst. The Ministry of Health (2002) reported that the frequency of uterine rupture in Guatemala is 1 out of every 1,500 to 2,000 pregnancies. The frequency of scar ruptures is even lower, as the reported number includes all causes of uterine rupture (e.g., car accidents, knife and gun wounds, congenital problems, etc.). The sheer likelihood of uterine rupture due to a previous c-section is so low that from 1996 to 2003 not one woman listed on the registry of maternal deaths in Sololá suffered one.

But the midwives' and families' reluctance to see their daughters and wives go to the hospital for a post-caesarean pregnancy ran even deeper. Delivering in the hospital might be less than ideal, but sending a woman off to be operated on again, they felt, was something to be avoided. The official policy in the Sololá hospital was updated in September 2002 to allow some women with c-section scars to try to deliver vaginally. So those who worked with the Safe Motherhood campaign made it clear that a woman with a scar who delivered in the hospital did not automatically have to have another c-section. Yet when I talked to people in the villages they insisted that if a woman with a scar was sent to the hospital, she would come home with another operation. I was sympathetic to women who did not want to go through another c-section unless it was absolutely necessary, and I had friends in the United States who went to "vaginal birth after caesarean section" birthing classes to try to avoid the same fate. So when I worked in the hospital I tried to understand why midwives, their clients, and families thought that going back to the hospital meant another c-section. What I found was though official policy might have changed, the conditions under which doctors worked didn't. This meant that most women would probably be subjected to another c-section automatically.

The official policy said that women who had horizontal incisions ("with the grain") in their uteruses were allowed to attempt a vaginal birth, while those whose uteruses that were cut vertically (against the "grain" and therefore cutting more muscles) would have to deliver by another c-section. What determined if a woman had been cut horizontally or vertically? The two gynecologists and three GPs that staffed the ER and did the surgeries told me that the horizontal cut is preferable precisely because the procedure is relatively less risky for subsequent births. Vertical incisions are, however, sometimes used because doctors said that it is easier to get a baby out of a vertical cut than out of a horizontal one. For example, it is sometimes difficult to find a foot and pull the baby out of the uterus if the baby is transverse.[6] A vertical incision guarantees a fast delivery no matter the position or the circumstances; so if time were of the essence, a vertical incision may have been used.

The change in official policy is unlikely to have had much effect on the number of vaginal deliveries after caesareans because it is difficult for attending physicians to ascertain if a patient's uterus was cut horizontally or vertically. First, most patients were never given the information about what sort of incision was used in their operation, and if they were it was unlikely that they understood or could remember. Second, most of the doctors in Sololá cut the external abdominal tissue vertically, leaving a scar from the belly button to the pubis. This scar, however, gives no information about the position of the scar inside on the uterus. Third, medical records for the procedure are only available if the woman had the previous operation in the Sololá hospital *and* if she has brought the file number that she was assigned during the previous procedure. Much to the chagrin of the Ministry of Health many patients lost track of or forgot their old hospital cards, so they got new patient numbers and started new files with every visit to the hospital. As some procedures demand vertical incisions rather than horizontal, doctors will usually ask the reason for a previous caesarean. The end result is that doctors can sometimes eliminate the possibility that a woman had a horizontal incision, but can never rule out a vertical. Erring on the side of caution means that if you don't know what kind of incision the c-section was, you should deliver by c-section. So, while the policy may have changed, the conditions of practice are such that most women who come through the door with a previous c-section scar were operated on.

Again, what this example shows us is that the Safe Motherhood campaign in Sololá was looking outward toward international experience and best biomedical protocol to establish their guidelines. Iyoma's understandings of pregnancy and birth, however, were firmly rooted in their experiences in Sololá. What the iyoma noticed was that there was a disjuncture between what the Safe Motherhood campaign said and what actually happened. The information that they were being taught about post-caesarean deliveries (first, that they should automatically deliver by caesarean for the next pregnancy, and later, that while they are dangerous, women will be allowed to try a vaginal delivery in the hospital) did not bear out. What could that say about the rest of the information that the Safe Motherhood campaign was trying to teach them? Why should the iyoma privilege knowledge that contradicted their own?

Authority and Biomedical Pluralism

Ironically, predicating the Safe Motherhood campaign on the latest biomedical knowledge concerning obstetrics created a context that made the information doubtful to iyoma in other ways. The Ministry of Health, and the NGOs that worked with it to run the campaign, assumed a special relationship to iyoma as *the* supplier of biomedical information, rather than *a* supplier of biomedical information. While in the past the Ministry of Health might not have had to contend for iyoma's attention with any competing biomedical providers, as transportation and communication have become cheaper, the quantity of healthcare options available to people in the health district have significantly increased.

As many villagers pointed out to me, relying on the public system wasn't always feasible. All three of the villages that I worked in had Ministry of Health buildings, yet one of the main complaints that I heard from men and women was that the auxiliary nurses who staffed the health posts weren't available frequently enough. The nurse only got paid to work from 8:00 AM to 4:30 PM, Monday through Friday,[7] and the post was closed a half day on Monday for an in-service meeting. Of the eighteen days a month that the health post was officially open the nurse did not attend patients for three of those days, while she was vaccinating.[8] Finally, the Ministry of Health gave auxiliary nurses thirty working days off per year, and though theoretically a substitute worker was supposed to fill in during the nurse's vacation, the district was never allotted enough money to maintain the surplus worker, so the health post remained closed during this time. Villagers also had the option of going to the health center in San Pablo or to the hospital in Sololá. Using the health center in San Pablo was not a popular option for Cruceños since it cost the same amount of time and money as going to the hospital in Sololá, yet it was less equipped.[9] In addition, one could take advantage of the trip to the hospital to also visit one of the largest markets in the area.[10]

Nevertheless, there were many other options for care that were more appealing. With the proliferation of cell phones and motor boats, going into "town" to contact a biomedical healthcare provider was now relatively easy. Midwives frequently formed relationships with certain doctors and/or pharmacists, in addition to auxiliary nurses and professional nurses. For example, Doña Berta reported that she accompanied all of her patients that she was worried about to a private doctor in San Pedro, because the wait with him was short. Like most doctors' offices in the area, patients were seen on a first come, first serve basis. Apparently this doctor had instructed his assistants to always move Doña Berta's clients to the front of the line. In an environment where many women complained that they were frequently treated unfairly and made to wait for care longer than others because they were outsiders (i.e., from a different town), this special treatment secured Doña Berta's continued patronage. The same sorts of relationships were rumored to be established between midwives and pharmacists.[11] Iyoma turned to the pharmacist to inform them about the latest drugs. Doctors at the hospital reported that through these channels some iyoma obtained quinine or Pitocin, which they used to hurry along a birth.

In addition to the host of local biomedical practitioners functioning outside of the State-provided care, iyoma also came into contact with a plethora of foreign doctors, nurses, and nurse-midwives and professional midwives who were also involved in imparting biomedical information. There were a number of foreign NGOs that recruited foreign doctors to donate a week of their time to conduct skills workshops for local midwives. The midwives frequently received graduation certificates or medical supplies such as gloves, scissors, food, or even a small daily stipend for their participation. In the health district that Santa Cruz is part of the midwives also availed themselves of a free clinic run by a US-trained nurse and professional midwife, who also accepted foreign-trained midwife volunteers from a variety of countries. This nurse worked in conjunction with a Dutch doctor, who was present in the clinic at least half of the year. She was very active in networking with iyoma and bolstering safe homebirth. In short, iyoma are anything but isolated from biomedical knowledge and providers.

The problem this created for the authority of the Safe Motherhood campaign was that the Ministry of Health and the NGOs that it partnered with had no control over and, in most cases, no data concerning the information other biomedical practitioners were teaching iyoma. Iyoma frequently received diametrically opposed advice from two different biomedical practitioners. For example, the pharmacist told them to use Pitocin, but the health workers affiliated with Safe Motherhood told them not to, and yet iyoma could observe the doctors in the hospital using it. In another example, in a Safe Motherhood training workshop on reducing post-partum hemorrhage through massage, an iyom questioned the form of the massage that we were learning. She had been to a workshop the week before led by Canadian doctors who taught her an entirely different method of massage. The instructor reviewed what she was doing and told her that the Canadian method had been incorrect, and what she was learning today would help her more. In another example, iyoma received mixed messages about breech births and twins. Officially, iyoma were to refer clients who present with either condition. The foreign professional midwives, however, told local iyoma that twins and breech births could easily be delivered safely at home and that there was no need for these clients to deliver in the hospital. They offered to accompany iyoma to these births as an alternative to transporting the birthing women.

From the perspectives of the iyoma, biomedical advice was variable across time as well as from provider to provider.[12] While the biomedical knowledge concerning what constitutes an obstetric emergency has remained relatively stable over time, policies concerning how to handle these emergencies change. The Safe Motherhood campaign was linked to international centers of public health that were involved in collating the most recent and contextually useful information necessary to decrease maternal mortality. Health workers at all levels routinely attended conferences to update their training.

From health workers' views, these changes in techniques, information, and policies spoke for the integrity of the campaign; for the iyoma the effect was just the opposite. The iyoma had little insight into why certain policies changed—why, for example, one week they officially could deliver breech births and the next week they could not. In their eyes, the fact that policies and information coming out of the Safe Motherhood effort were not set in stone made the campaign seem more negotiable and arbitrary rather than more valid.

In sum, while health workers might feel confident in the superior reliability of scientifically grounded information, from the iyoma's perspectives the "official" biomedical protocols that they were taught were quite compromised. These protocols frequently contradicted iyoma's own experiences, different biomedical practitioners gave diametrically opposed advice about the same problem, and policies were continually changing—all factors that collaborated to undermine the authority of the Safe Motherhood campaign as a good font of information. Iyoma did not know nor understand the difference in training between a GP, an OB, a professional midwife, a professional nurse, a nurse practitioner, and a pharmacist, foreign or locally trained. They were not evaluating the knowledge from the perspective of its scientific validity. Instead, as Doña Berta's example showed, many of the iyoma's own choices concerning biomedical healthcare providers were made by prioritizing trust between the provider and the iyom herself.[13] The challenge of obtaining referrals might be partially predicated on didactic methods and midwife understanding, but perhaps the larger challenge is securing the respect and trust of the iyoma in order to ensure their cooperation.

Why Women Don't Go to the Hospital

I met Florinda one April morning while interviewing women in her village about pregnancy-related emergencies and their feelings about going to the hospital. As we talked about her reproductive history she told me that her first baby was stillborn. Her second pregnancy went much better; the delivery itself was relatively easy and she gave birth to a healthy baby boy. Later in the interview I returned to Florinda's two birth experiences, but this time I let the Safe Motherhood campaign's definitions of problems during birth guide my questions. When I asked her if she had ever had to wait more than thirty minutes for the placenta to come out, she told me that with the second birth she did—in fact, she waited two hours. According to the Safe Motherhood campaign's guidelines Florinda should have been transported to the hospital for emergency obstetric care, lest she bleed to death.

Florinda herself was firm about going to the hospital if she ever had an obstetric emergency. Interestingly, however, she would not go to the hospital if this same thing happened to her again. In no part of the interview did she identify the retention of her placenta for two hours as an obstetric emergency. Instead, to show that it had just been a delay, she pointed to the fact that it *had* come out and that she was doing fine. Even when she agreed with me that retaining the placenta for two hours was not exactly normal and that her mother and mother-in-law were worried, she disagreed that what had happened to her was an emergency. An emergency, she felt, was a birthing problem that could not be resolved. Looking back, it was obvious that her problem had been resolved. So she disagreed that the proper way to deal with what happened to her was to go to the hospital.

Why would women who were willing to go to the hospital not be willing to use the guidelines on which the Safe Motherhood campaign based its referrals? Florinda's case is typical of birth stories women told me and illustrative of women's perceptions that the Safe Motherhood guidelines could not be used to actually identify birthing emergencies. The guidelines mixed all women together as if they were the same, but, as interviewees and iyoma told me over and over again, every woman is different. Some women had babies easily while others suffered through every minute of pregnancy and labor. Some women got pregnant over and over again while others only had three or four children. Some women birthed the placenta immediately while it took others longer.[14]

Not only is every woman distinct, but the Kaqchikel women whom I interviewed saw the likelihood of a problem or complication in pregnancy or birth as pegged to individual circumstances and characteristics. Whether or not a birth was problematic was linked to relationships within the community. Rosario's death, which began this book, highlights this framework. If someone had a vendetta against you, your husband, or either of your families, they could hex your birth. Despite the fact that Evangelicals and iyoma have foresworn contact with the bad powers and spirits, witchcraft was still seen as a common source of birthing problems.[15] More transparent relationship problems were also held to blame. Sandra told me that one of her births had taken more than five days. Why did it take so long, I asked? Probably, she said, because she had been fighting a lot with her sisters-in-law during the pregnancy. As the birth is a family event, if things are not going well within the family, they might not go well within the birth. A bad relationship between a husband and wife, the central actors in the birth narrative, can be the root of even worse problems. Husbands who don't take care of their wives and fight a lot with their wives while they are pregnant were also blamed for causing birthing problems.

But a pregnant woman's own behavior could also have serious consequences for her delivery. Pregnant woman should not work too much while they are pregnant. They should give up collecting firewood, which involves walking long distances up mountainous terrain and carrying extremely heavy loads on their backs. They should not work in the fields. They should try to relax. A woman who did not respect her pregnancy, and therefore did not respect herself, was deemed irresponsible because she knew that she could be provoking problems. But pregnancy also challenged a woman spiritually. Being at odds with God, either by doubting your own faith or by sinning (having an affair, drinking, or somehow cheating someone) could put you at risk for a difficult pregnancy.[16]

There were also crucial choices that a family had to make in relation to a pregnancy or birth that was perceived to involve risk. Doña Cecilia, one of the oldest iyoma working in Santa Cruz, basically stopped attending births during my second year of fieldwork. The rumors were that no one wanted to go to her. Three of her last four deliveries had complications—one of which resulted in Rosario's death. While some people suggested that the births were complicated by the fates of the delivering women themselves, others argued that it was Doña Cecilia who was cursed. She could have been cursed by a specific person or she could have been cursed in the spiritual realm. Either way, many women who had been delivered by her in the past did not deliver with her again. Families that switched iyoma were being proactive and protecting themselves by staving off potential problems in upcoming births.[17]

This understanding of risk that many birthing families and their iyoma held created an intractable difference with the Safe Motherhood campaign's guidelines.[18] The guidelines were based on research that crunched population-level data to try to distinguish the bounds of normal from abnormal. For example, most women's placentas will come out within thirty minutes. While not all who have to wait more than thirty minutes will experience problems, we don't know who will have a problem and who won't. The cause of the problem is, therefore, imagined to be random. The important point is that if all of the women whose placentas were retained for more than thirty minutes went to the hospital immediately, they would almost certainly arrive in time for the doctors to take care of a problem *if it did* arise. In the end, no one would have to die from a retained placenta. Yet this sort of system was not amenable to most people in Santa Cruz. They did not see obstetric problems and complications as random, but rather as directly tied to their own relationships. Since families and iyoma perceived social aspects of their situation as determinant, they believed that they had much more control over their own vulnerability than biomedicine would assign. In essence, a family with a clean conscience might be prone to wait several hours for a placenta to come out, while one that had not been so fortunate might not.

The goal of the Safe Motherhood campaign, to make sure that no woman who *could* be saved instead dies, also meant that many women whose complications would resolve themselves if given time were asked to go to or birth in the hospital. Health workers viewed the extra hospital deliveries as an almost negligible cost. Indeed, the costs themselves were only ever talked about in terms of money. As I discussed in the first chapter, however, going to the hospital obviated very important and irreplaceable opportunities to integrate the family. In addition, for women and their families, going to the hospital involved a number of unacknowledged costs that made it the last option.

Unacknowledged Costs of Using the Hospital

Ana Emiliana was one of the first women I interviewed in the ER who had not wanted to come to the hospital. She was admitted with a terrible post-partum infection. She had given birth several days beforehand and now had a swollen abdomen, a high fever, and was issuing putrid smells. She was very weak and had become delirious. Her family had waited several days for her symptoms to clear up, but when her fever persisted and she seemed to get worse rather than better they decided to take her to the ER.

When I encountered Ana Emiliana she was begging me to help her leave the hospital. After she had been rushed in by her family members the nurse asked them to change her and then leave. The nurse started Ana Emiliana on an antibiotic drip and then told her that she would have to wait for the doctor. I sat in the corner of the room taking notes and observing. The nurse had not closed Ana Emiliana's shower curtain, so she saw me in the room. Since I was not wearing a health workers' uniform, almost no patients or their family members took note of me or talked to me while I was in the ER. But Ana Emiliana specifically called to me and asked me to come to her bed. When I got there she told me that her family had left her, but that she needed to leave the hospital now lest she die here. She said that she would not be able to survive alone and was very afraid of what would happen to her if forced to stay. I told her that she was sick and that she had been brought to the hospital for a cure. I asked her to wait for the doctor. She repeated that she needed to leave. She didn't care what the doctor said, there was no way she was going to spend the night in the hospital all alone. I told her that she would go to the women's ward, where only women with problems like hers slept. There were six beds in the room. They had a bathroom and the hospital would give her food. She told me that if her family left her here they would operate on her and that she would not survive an operation. Ana Emiliana was desperate. She was crying. She was clutching my hand and either trying to pull herself up or pull me down to her. We talked for a few minutes while she waited for the doctor. I eventually promised her that I would go to the women's ward with her, check in on her before I left the hospital that day, and visit her every morning to see how she was doing. While I did not really have anything else to offer her, she had little choice but to stay and be comforted by my company. I visited her the next morning in the hospital and she agreed that she was not scared anymore and felt much better. After several days of being fed antibiotics through an IV solution, Ana Emiliana's fever had completely disappeared, her infection had cleared up, and she went home.

What happened to Ana Emiliana is an excellent illustration of how terrified women and their families were of using the hospital. People had a number of reasons why they were afraid to go. If a woman were forced to labor and birth without her family members, who would see to her needs? Who would be there to take care of her after the birth?[19] Finally, many women stressed their own fear of being in a hospital where they could not speak the same language as the healthcare providers. What if someone asked you something and you answered wrong and they gave you the wrong treatment? What if they asked you if you wanted to be operated on and you didn't understand enough to say "no?" And what if you needed something, but no one could understand what it was? While these items were not mentioned as reasons *not* to go to the hospital if you absolutely had to, they undoubtedly represent costs that make women reluctant to go until the last minute.

While Ana Emiliana told me all of this, what I have tried to get across in her narrative is the extra pain that one must feel confronting these things when one is already half near death. It was the desperation and fear that was often missing when I described my work to friends, neighbors or acquaintances after I had finished my fieldwork and returned to Michigan. Many found it absolutely mindboggling that someone would be so reluctant to go to the hospital that they would rather chance dying. It just seemed too counterintuitive. Yet in the post-9/11 world in which I was working on this manuscript, I finally came up with an apt comparison to get across to my friends and relatives what a woman and her family might feel like. I told them, imagine you, a US citizen, are alone in a village in Afghanistan and you (or your wife or sister) are giving birth and have a problem. Your only option is a Taliban controlled hospital and you don't speak any local languages. If you go there, people have told you that you will be separated from your family and not permitted to be accompanied by anyone. Can you imagine the terror of such a choice? Can you imagine how you would feel being left in an enemy hospital in such a vulnerable state?[20]

In this section I explain why women and their families turned to the hospital as their last choice. The most oft-repeated problem was a fear of a caesarean section. While antibiotics, IVs, X-rays, and ultrasounds were all extremely popular biomedical technologies in Sololá, any technologies that were based on cutting the body or removing fluids were equally unpopular. Accordingly, autopsies, blood donation, and operations were generally eschewed. Unfortunately, these procedures were frequently associated with obstetric emergencies.[21]

"Operations"

Operations have no parallels in "traditional" medicine that Kaqchikel villagers use, and on an intuitive level it is not difficult to understand why they are so unpopular. Cutting a body open seems inherently invasive and dangerous, and it is difficult to imagine that anyone weak, sick, or compromised could have the strength to survive such an ordeal. To add insult to injury the chronic shortage of blood for a patient who needs an operation is a constant recurrent theme in Guatemala. The official Ministry of Health policy is that no one in need will be denied an operation due to a lack of blood, yet the hospital system is always in need of more blood. What I witnessed, as I describe in Cristina's story below, is that operations frequently turned into battles for blood donation between the hospital staff and the family of a sick person.

Cristina was a young woman and it was rumored that she had had an affair with a married man from another town. She came home sick and was bedridden. Some claimed that she had sought out an illegal abortion, but after two weeks her family took her to the Sololá hospital saying that she had been bleeding from the anus. By the time that she was admitted she was so weak that she could not walk. From the moment she arrived the hospital staff began to tell the family how imperative it was to Cristina's health that they donate blood. They tested my husband, who had accompanied them to the ER, and the two family members present. My husband was rejected as a potential donor since he did not have Cristina's blood type, and no one gave blood that afternoon. In between fretting over Cristina's state her family spent the next two days asking everyone they knew to donate blood for Cristina and worrying that she was going to die if she didn't get it. After Cristina's condition did not improve her doctors in Sololá transferred her to a hospital in Guatemala City so that she could have an endoscopy (not available in Sololá). During the week that she waited for the endoscopy the whole question of blood donation evaporated. After the endoscopy failed to reveal the source of the hemorrhage and Cristina was scheduled for exploratory surgery, however, it resurfaced with a fury. When we talked to her brother he seemed to believe that her life *depended* on receiving the blood. Thus, I drew the conclusion that perhaps if the hospital didn't get the donation, they wouldn't do the operation or give Cristina any transfusions. Since her family was still talking about blood type it seemed as if any blood gathered was going to go directly to her.

Cristina's brother, Eduardo, decided to go back to Guatemala City to give blood (which up to this point he had not done), but volunteers to accompany him were few. Neither my husband nor I could go on the designated day. We did, however, hang up a sign in one of the tourist hotels, hoping to find a backpacker who didn't mind visiting the hospital for a day. Jerry, a Dutch lawyer, volunteered to go and the next day he and Eduardo traveled to the hospital in Guatemala City. Jerry unfortunately passed out as he attempted to donate and was, therefore, rejected. He then related to us that he had attempted to pay a taxi driver waiting outside of the hospital to give blood, but the taxi driver said that he couldn't because he had eaten meat in the morning. Through Jerry we learned that an individual's blood type was no longer relevant. In addition, Jerry brought the question to head, would the hospital give Cristina blood if there are no donors? Through the two weeks of treatment no one had asked that question and no one in the hospital had volunteered the information. We visited an auxiliary nurse who had worked in the health system for twenty years and she explained that the hospital would not let Cristina die for lack of donors.

After the exploratory surgery, the hospital really started to push the family for more and more donors. Her brother was frantic, more convinced than ever that if he did not find more donors for Cristina that her condition would deteriorate even more. I called the hospital in Guatemala City to make an appointment to donate blood for Cristina and was put on hold. When the operator answered she told me that Cristina was very weak and that it was, therefore, imperative that they receive blood donations now. She urged me to come as soon as possible. She then transferred me to Cristina's room where her second brother was visiting her. He answered the phone and instantly began urging me to come and give blood. He told me that Cristina was not doing well. At this point it became clear to me that there was little causal relationship between blood donations and Cristina's condition. She had already had surgery. She was receiving blood from a bank, not from direct donors. Yet the hospital staff was downplaying these facts and intentionally or unintentionally, the message that the family was receiving was that Cristina's condition and eventual recovery was intimately tied to her receiving more blood.

The next day my husband went back to talk to the retired nurse who had just returned from the hospital in Guatemala City. She told him that not one of Cristina's family members had donated blood for her. To date, the hospital had received only one pint in her name. Asking Cristina's family members why they had not given blood was not a neutral question. They were at least outwardly convinced that much of her fate hung on their ability to procure donations. They had asked my husband and me to give. It would be a very delicate matter to tell us why they couldn't also do it. Nevertheless, I felt that it was important to ask. Eduardo, her first brother, had paid 300 Q, a quarter of his monthly salary, to an acquaintance to travel to the hospital and donate blood. Eduardo said that he had tried to give but that the hospital refused to take his blood because he had a fungus on his fingers or toes. Cristina's other two brothers, both of whom had been to see her, had less articulate answers. Keylor said that he had no blood to give. David didn't want to answer the question.

When I was on the boat heading to the catch the bus to the city in order to donate blood, Ada, an acquaintance sitting next to me, struck up a conversation. When I told her that I was going to the city she immediately asked me if I was going to see Cristina; I told her that actually I was going to give blood. She then began asking me about what they did when they took your blood. I told her. She said that people in Santa Cruz work hard all day and, therefore, can't give blood. They need their strength and can't risk that they might faint. I emphasized several times that there were no lasting effects from giving blood, but she kept returning to the point, what if you faint while giving blood? I told her that I thought that people were just scared, but she emphasized that they just could not risk fainting.

As this example illustrates, operations are dreaded cures not only because of their objectionable qualities, but because operations intertwine the fate of your loved one with your own corporeal sacrifice. Regardless of the specific beliefs underwriting Keylor and Ada's articulated responses to giving blood, they did not view giving blood as a benign activity for the donor, but rather as potentially injurious. This viewpoint is certainly shored up by the general lack of food available to people and the extreme physical demands of daily work for both women and men. It is also concurrent with widespread beliefs from the Andes to Tanzania that blood is a non-renewable resource, and thus removal of blood will leave you weak (Allen 2002; Bastien 1985).

In addition to the potential physical cost of donating, Weismantel (2001) and Scheper-Hughes (1996) highlight the metaphor of extraction that could make blood donation appear dangerous. The poor throughout Latin America worry about those who are more powerful extracting bodily products from them. Bob Simpson (2009) also argues the ability of a State or political group to voluntarily receive blood donations from its public is a mark of its legitimacy. For Guatemala, then, perhaps the refusal to donate is also read by hospital staff as a tacit allegation of the illegitimacy of the post-war State. Perhaps the inability of the Ministry of Health to procure blood speaks again to the fissure between itself and the population of poor, indigenous citizens who it purports to serve. Faced with an inability to procure blood voluntarily, the Ministry of Health must depend on "forcible and immoral extraction" (Simpson 2009:115). Despite the fact the policy of donation was officially voluntary hospital staff obviously pressured family members (if not patients themselves) for blood. Alice Street (2009) shows how such an approach to blood donation can further alienate the patient in the hospital from the services they seek.

Toward the end of my second year of fieldwork this issue of blood donation exploded again, but this time in Tzununá, one of the other villages that I worked in. The nurse in the village told me that a woman, Constancia, who was eight months pregnant had arrived to the health post on a Friday to seek treatment because she was spotting blood. The nurse examined her and found that the spotting wasn't very heavy, so she told Constancia that she was fine. On Monday, Constancia's husband came back to the health post and said that Constancia was in bed, bleeding, and couldn't get up. The nurse went to examine Constancia again and saw a large pool of blood in her bed. The nurse told the husband that unless they went to the hospital immediately, Constancia would die. Constancia and her husband then hitched a ride with the police to the hospital in Sololá, where the doctors gave her blood and delivered the baby via caesarean section. Constancia had been diagnosed with a condition called placenta previa, where the placenta is wedged between the cervix and uterus, instead of above the uterus. The pressure of the uterus on the placenta caused a rupture that led to continued bleeding. Both Constancia and her baby, however, were fine. But then a doctor or a nurse went after the family and told them that they had to take four blood donors to Guatemala City at that moment to replace the blood that was used to save Constancia. The family felt that they were being threatened. Regardless of whether or not this family was reluctant to give blood, going to Guatemala City represented both a significant amount of money in transport costs (about two days' wages per person) and danger, as villagers make easy targets for thieves. Finally, the situation was de-escalated because the family went and talked to the hospital social worker, who was there to help families cover exorbitant medical costs (like going to Guatemala City). After hearing the story, the social worker accompanied the family back to the staff member in question and confronted him or her. The social worker advised the staff member that s/he had no right to be putting so much pressure on the family, or making demands that they travel to the city immediately. Once back in Tzununá, the husband emphasized to the local nurse that he got Constancia and the baby out of the hospital as soon as possible. Constancia and her husband then told everyone in the village not to go to the hospital because the staff will threaten you and try to steal your blood. Despite the fact that Constancia and her baby were saved, the visit to the hospital was a fiasco.

The insistence that family replace blood used by a patient is an instance of staff picking and choosing which global health protocols they will promote and which they let fall by the wayside. The WHO has rejected the policy of asking kin to replace blood, yet estimates that the majority of all blood collected in developing countries is either donated by the family or procured by paying a donor (World Health Organization 2005). At first glance it is difficult to understand the actions of the hospital staff, who promote the dated system of coercing patients to give blood, and who intentionally misrepresent how blood is apportioned throughout the health system. On the other hand, obligating blood donation can be also be read as an attempt to educate patients about appropriate participation, as discussed in chapter 4. By giving blood, patients support the healing of the post-war national body.[22]

Though caesarean section, the most common surgery associated with emergency obstetric care, does not usually involve blood donation, women and their families also tried to avoid this procedure at all possible costs. During interviews, women emphasized that caesareans were major operations and one never knew if a woman would hold on and endure or just die on the operating table. Women's own c-section scars reinforced their idea of the enormity of the operation. Unlike in North America, where most women receive small incisions that are easily hidden by a bikini, in Sololá most of the incisions were quite large. As many doctors told me, since Mayan women were not in the practice of wearing bikinis, what the scar looked like after the operation was considered a minor concern. While no woman I talked to ever referred to any cosmetic aspect of these scars, many referred to the relationship between the size of the scar, its place, and the major nature of the surgery.

Dinora's story illustrates this. My field assistant, Isabel, and I had just finished completing an interview with Dinora and were getting ready to go when she said that she wanted to talk to us about another topic. She told us that she was having a problem with her uterus, and that it was not staying put. It was obvious from what she said that she had a prolapsed uterus, a condition where the womb falls down and can begin to come out of the vagina. She wanted to know how to get it fixed. Having been through this with another woman, I knew the procedure well. I told her that she would have to go to the obstetrician at the hospital, be diagnosed, have a few tests, and then they would operate on her and remove her uterus.

She was very adamant that she was not going to be operated on to cure herself of this problem. She'd rather keep the problem and live than risk the operation and potential death.

Isabel and I left, and as we walked we talked about prolapsed uteruses. In the conversation I mentioned that the doctors go in through the vagina and cut the uterus out so there is no external scar on the abdomen. Isabel came to a complete stop and exclaimed with surprise that the surgery was not so major after all. I said that I thought that it was not minor, since they removed an organ from your body. Regardless of what they took, Isabel said, they don't cut through your body to get it. Therefore, she said, the surgery was not major. She said that we should have told Dinora that information and that maybe then she would feel differently about fixing her prolapse.

Women's reluctance to have caesarean sections goes even further than their general reluctance to have a major operation. Several of my informal conversations alerted me to the fact that women were potentially confusing tubal ligations with caesarean deliveries. Lexically, both procedures were known as "operation." Though in the hospital, Spanish-speaking health workers employ the technical word *cesárea*, outside of the hospital Spanish-speaking lay people only used *operación* or referred to being operated on (*me operaron*). The same means were employed to express that a woman had had a tubal ligation. I never heard any Kaqchikel term for either c-section or tubal ligation. Instead, women employed the Spanish term and said *nub'än operación* (to do operation) or *nub'än operar* (to operate).

My data support the argument that the lack of a lexical distinction between the two procedures has created confusion among women about exactly what a caesarean section involves, and, more importantly, how it affects their fertility. In my formal interviews, I asked women: In your opinion, if they operate on a woman in the hospital for problems with her delivery, will it hurt her ability to have more children? Of the 90 women who I asked the question, 60 percent (54) believed that the woman's ability to have children would be negatively affected, 18 percent (16) said that they didn't know, and 19 percent (17) thought that the c-section would not affect future childbearing. I do not want to argue that my data definitely show that all of the women who said "yes" do not understand that there are two different procedures; it was impossible to ask that question without biasing the answer. What I would argue is that the conflation of tubal ligation and caesarean by some women stimulates a discourse of the negative effect of a c-section on a woman's ability to have more children. Some women who had not had c-sections heard the question and then reasoned that the woman a few houses up had a c-section and she had had more children, so no, c-sections did not hurt. Yet, other women who had delivered by c-section answered that c-sections did hurt your ability to have more children. They said that c-sections made it harder for them to get pregnant and harder for them to deliver. The Safe Motherhood campaign's own guidelines that a woman with a previous c-section should deliver in the hospital was interpreted by respondents as supporting the contention that c-sections made it harder to birth subsequent babies.

The danger to your fertility of getting a caesarean in a public hospital if you were indigenous is perhaps most poignantly demonstrated by the following story. One of the Ministry of Health doctors told me that there were rumors during the civil war that doctors responsible for operating on indigenous women frequently performed tubal ligations if it was feasible. Each tubal ligation was performed under the slogan "one less guerilla." As far as I know there is no evidence of a campaign of forced sterilization of indigenous women in Guatemala. However, the story does underscore the ethnic and political differences between some doctors who work(ed) for the Ministry of Health and the indigenous clientele that they serve. It also reveals why women and their families might have be reluctant to seek out an emergency c-section if they would be operated on by someone whom they could not trust.

Lawrence Cohen's (2003) interviews with individuals in the Indian "kidney belt," where villagers in need of money frequently are reduced to selling their organs, highlight some of the particular concerns that operations can trigger for the poor. The scar can stand as indelible evidence of poverty—in Cohen's case people sold their kidneys to pay for costs incurred in their everyday lives. In Guatemala, women who use the public hospital for birth are distinguished by their particularly large abdominal scars. Like donating blood, operations were seen as procedures that could test the limits of the body. In India, women said that they had undergone operations because their husbands needed strength to work. Operations could sap the vigor out of bodies needed for physical labor. In Guatemala, women and the families also worried about the toll that the operation could take on a body, especially while the surgery was being conducted.

For the Safe Motherhood campaign and the Ministry of Health, the fact that an emergency obstetric procedure and a family-planning

procedure have the same name is quite unfortunate. Forced sterilization or control of fertility in minority and indigenous populations through the guise of public health initiatives has a long history
(Ralstin-Lewis 2005; Torpy 2000; Lawrence 2000). The Kaqchikel
villages where I worked were extremely pronatalist and family planning was contentious. Women and their families worried about the
effects of an operation on their fertility. As Caroline Bledsoe (2002)
described, women seemed to view fertility as a limited resource and
having an operation could use up a part of them (forever). Less metaphorically, women worried about what would happen to their productive capacity while they went under the knife. Cecilia Van Hollen
(2003) vividly describes how health workers in India "maneuver[ed]
development during the post-partum period"—meaning that they
routinely inserted IUDs into patients to make sure that State-wide
goals for contraception were met. The Ministry of Health was very
much identified with the national family planning campaign and
was seen as eager to limit fertility. Women and their families feared
that if they went to the public hospital for a c-section, they might
come out unable to have more babies.

Religious Costs of Using the Hospital

The increased importance of Evangelical religion in Santa Cruz aug-
mented the costs of seeking emergency obstetric care in the hospital.
Evangelical churches were local institutions and were intertwined
with local power politics in a way that Catholicism was not. While
Catholics at all levels were subject to the interloping of senior church
authorities, Evangelicals could organize as many followers as possible, with little or no outside interference.[23] Being a pastor was a reflection of one's high social status in the village and evidence of one's
influence. Accordingly, the formation of Evangelical churches in Santa
Cruz tended to be driven by personal power politics more than ideological religious differences. Two of the four Evangelical churches
were formed when church leaders fought with one another, which
resulted in a separation of congregations into factions. The fourth
was recently formed when a former mayor decided to build his own
church, principally as evidence of his status.

Because the differences between local churches graph more closely
onto cleavages between local power factions than onto any real religious differences, I would argue that "branding the church" is an
important part of consolidating power. By "branding" I mean to suggest that certain practices are deemed contraband to give identity to
a congregation rather than to differentiate ideologies. In one con-

versation, a Cruceño made reference to the fact that in the Bible God said that men had to wear pants and women had to wear skirts. When I asked him in what part of the Bible that was written, he said that he didn't know, but that his pastor had imposed that rule on the congregation so that they would follow what the Lord said. In another church, I found out that the pastor forbid women from wearing beaded necklaces. Perhaps more directly related to my work, one pastor forbade parishioners from seeking outside help or being involved in non-religious institutions or organizations. In general, he refused to enter into a dialogue with civic or development organizations and initiatives. His ostensible reasoning was that he was a man of God and religion. He, therefore, restricted himself to religious activity. He did not see the improvement of the water system, the evacuation of obstetric emergencies from the village, or the distribution of food goods to children as related to the religious domain. He encouraged his parishioners to stay within the religious domain, be pious, and trust God's will. Rather than seeking biomedical interventions, he asked instead that members rely on prayer and God's power to cure themselves.

Going against these edicts could be quite costly. In evangelical churches the idea that what you learned in church should be practiced at home was not implicit; it was enforced.[24] Atonement in the evangelical church was a public process. The sins of evangelical congregants became a topic of worship discussions. To atone, congregants not only should publicly ask for forgiveness from the congregation, but sinners in an evangelical church could be punished. They could lose special privileges that marked their status in the church, such as their right to go and worship in the church unattended, whenever they felt the need. They could lose the congregation's trust. They could be forced to sit at the back of the church. All of these penalties marked a diminished status in the church and, correspondingly, among one's social peers. Sinners could recoup their status by being pious and not sinning again, and then could be forgiven. Religion was a yardstick applied to their own lives by their families, other congregants, and, most importantly, the pastor.[25]

Evangelic churches were so active that membership in the church could organize daily life. The population of the village was small and families were large, so one was constantly going to church to attend a funeral, baptism, confirmation, marriage, or some other event. Prayer was an important part of religious practice and every morning one woke to the sound of fellow congregation members greeting the new day over a portable loudspeaker. Walking though the village one frequently heard the chanting of a group of women, either convening on their own or participating in a prayer intervention, pouring out from a house onto the street. Everyday mechanisms to shun and punish any sin were bountiful, and that made the decision to transgress the pastor's wishes all the more difficult.

While normal use of the health post, hospital, or a doctor was frowned upon in this particular pastor's congregation, availing one's self of emergency obstetric care was a particularly egregious offense. As discussed in chapter 1, there was a strong relationship between iyoma, pregnancy, birth, and religion. Iyoma were chosen and trained through divine inspiration and both the fetus and its destiny were created by God. As birth was viewed as the outgrowth of God's will, having problems in one's birth was frequently interpreted as evidence of a disruption in a birthing woman's relationship with God.[26] Seeking biomedical care (and thereby publicly validating the disruption's existence) was socially quite costly for an evangelical woman and her family in this congregation.

Indeed, the discourse produced in this church had become so dominant in the village that birth had become a test. A woman and her family whose faith in God was secure and whose behavior was above reproach should have no difficulties. Though birthing problems were recognized to be both physiological and spiritual, the correct way to solve a problem was through prayer. Going to the hospital was tantamount to admitting a lack of faith in God. For families who were part of this congregation the social pressure not to use emergency obstetric care from the hospital and, thereby, not to jeopardize their standing in their religious community was strong. For families who were not part of the congregation they knew that seeking emergency medical care would foment rumors about their own religious conviction.

Lucrecia's experience directly illustrates this point. Lucrecia, a mother of six, sent for me through her sister. I had heard that she had had an extended labor, but word was that she had finally delivered the baby in the wee hours of Thursday morning. The baby was stillborn and had probably asphyxiated during the perilous labor. On Monday, five days after the birth, I pushed my way through a group of people milling about the courtyard of Lucrecia's family's compound. Lucrecia herself was in a one room adobe house in the back of the compound, accompanied by her older daughters, four sisters, and iyom. When I finally reached her I was shocked by her appearance. She looked more like a homunculus than the shy, amused, slight woman who sold Guatemalan weavings to tourists. Not only

was Lucrecia bundled from head to toe in blankets and bulky clothing, but the parts of her body that I could see—her hands and her
face—were incredibly bloated. She was completely conscious and I
bent down beside her and asked her how she felt. She said that she
was in extreme pain. She told me that the baby had been born dead,
but that it and placenta had come out fine. After the birth she never
recovered her strength, but just got worse. She told me that she
called me because she wanted to go to the hospital.

At this point her iyom, Ofelia, said that she had gone to see the
nurse earlier in the day. When Ofelia told Sofia, the nurse, about
Lucrecia's sickness, Sofia said that she got an infection from the caesarean scar that Lucrecia had from her last delivery. Ofelia said that
if we took Lucrecia to the hospital that they would have to clean
out her scar. She emphasized several times that they were going to
operate on Lucrecia if we took her to the hospital. I asked Ofelia if
the scar had ripped during Lucrecia's delivery and she said no. It
seemed to me that Ofelia was wielding the operation to advertise
the complete lunacy of taking a woman in Lucrecia's condition to
the hospital.[27] From her perspective Lucrecia was already weak and
an operation would have a good chance of killing her. Though Lucrecia and one of her sisters were in favor of going to the hospital,
none of the rest of her sisters or her midwife was in agreement. Her
husband was not in the village, but Lucrecia's daughter told me that
he had called and wanted her to go to the hospital. I told Lucrecia
that she had an infection which meant that in the hospital they
would give her antibiotics to kill the dirt and bugs in her blood. If
they needed to clean her scar, they could do it from the inside, and
if her placenta and baby were already out, they would not need to
operate. She said that she wanted to go, so I went and found transport and we left.

The fallout from Lucrecia's evacuation had begun as soon as she
left home. During visiting hours the day after, her husband stood
up and began a speech about how people were talking poorly about
them because Lucrecia had come to the hospital. "They" were saying that "we" don't trust or believe in God. But, he argued, God gave
doctors science and knowledge and so if Lucrecia gets an infection,
then God wants a doctor to see her and treat her. Why would they
stay at home and die if they could get treatment? He said that people
could say whatever they wanted, but it didn't bother him as long as
they were alive.

The retired nurse from the village, Laura, followed Lucrecia's husband and took up the defense. Laura said that she had gone and told

Ofelia off. Ofelia, she felt, was always the same—never listening to anyone else and never alerting anyone to a problem. Laura blamed this on Ofelia's own mistaken religious conviction. Laura, who was evangelical but attended a church outside of the village, said that she too believed in God, but that we are not so ensconced in God's good graces that we can hope that he will save us from everything. We have to take action ourselves.

Up to this point, I don't think that I had realized how much of a problem going to the hospital for an obstetric emergency could create for women and their families. While I don't think that anyone actively wanted a woman to die, there were definitely bitter differences about how exactly to go about saving someone in trouble. After the rather strong performances at the hospital I went back to talk to Ofelia. I was particularly interested in how she would respond to me after I took Lucrecia to the hospital. Ofelia was quite hospitable and grateful to receive the news that Lucrecia was out of danger.

Lucrecia's trouble helped me understand how social relationships in a sense controlled her fate. As Lucrecia birthed in her house her older daughters and sisters surrounded her for support. The younger children who gathered around the compound carried messages to those sister's husbands, and to me, keeping us informed about what was going on. When there were problems people were mobilized to pray. Though Lucrecia survived the birth, she was not out of trouble. Some of her sisters and her midwife wanted her to ride the infection out. She, her older daughters, and her sister, whose husband worked in the compound I lived in, wanted her to go to the hospital. I was called because Lucrecia had gotten stuck. No one was willing to take action and inertia would keep her home. I think that the main stumbling block was that her husband was not there. If he really wanted her to go to the hospital, why didn't he drop everything and come home? He was a powerful and mercurial man—no one wanted to cross him. Getting Lucrecia to the hospital was like moving through glue. Try as I might I could not delegate any tasks. I had to walk to a boat driver's house, negotiate the price of the boat, find the owner of the car, negotiate the price of the ride, find someone to call an ambulance to meet us, etc. When I visited Ofelia the next day I thought that due to her resistance she might be mad at me. I learned that she was far more diplomatic; she obviously felt that she had as much to lose by getting angry with me as I felt that I had to lose by getting angry with her.

Contextualizing Why Women Stay Home

When I came to Sololá, health workers had pointed out to me the inherent conflict that they saw between the strength of culture and traditions on the one hand, and a lack of dependence on hospital resources for obstetric emergencies on the other. The cost of breaking tradition seemed to be understood by them as an inertia cost, i.e., the more that you do things one way, the more likely you are to continue to do them that way. Yet, looking closer I found that the role of tradition or culture in shaping women's decisions concerning emergency obstetric care was not one of inertia, but was instead based on evaluating the costs and benefits of action in a particular circumstance. As I point out in chapter 1, while an older woman with seven or eight children might arguably be more steeped in the tradition of homebirth than a young married woman having her first child, seeking emergency obstetric care for the younger woman will incur more social costs.

In this chapter I have outlined many of the circumstances that motivate iyoma not to recommend emergency obstetric care, and many women and their families not to access those resources. The Safe Motherhood campaign's intervention was predicated on iyoma prioritizing information imparted in classes, without providing them any concrete experience or evidence that this information was helpful. In particular, there was a lack of focus on building relationships with iyoma practicing in the village. Yet, trust between health workers and iyoma was perhaps more paramount to the effectiveness of any policy concerning obstetric emergency than that policy's own scientific validity.

While the Safe Motherhood campaign prefers that women turn to biomedical emergency obstetric care as a first line of defense, this recommendation underestimates the actual social costs of using emergency obstetric care for women and their families. Procedures that health workers viewed as necessary and life-saving, women and their families viewed as risky and dangerous to a woman's own health and to her fertility. There was no reason to expose a woman to that risk and danger as a first line of defense. Moreover, transporting a woman to the hospital to resolve her obstetric problems frequently brought a woman and her family into conflict with a local, evangelical understanding of God's will. Seeking care then could jeopardize a woman and her families' social/religious status, and, perhaps more importantly, their own perceived relationship with

God. And even if a woman and her family were to disagree with this doctrine, by going to the hospital she and her family would have to suffer the gossip of neighbors. In short, going to the hospital for a birthing-related problem could be anathema to the social lives of women and their families. Nevertheless, as indicated in this chapter, sometimes families did exhaust all of their other options and felt that there was no better alternative but to go.

In this chapter we have also been able to see many of the everyday ways that the Safe Motherhood campaign encourages women and iyoma to privilege an understanding of birth as physiological process, and therefore encourages an understanding of birthing-related problems that is, likewise, physiological. For example, women and iyoma are taught simple rules to differentiate acceptable from unacceptable risk. These rules assume the existence of a universal, female person that is common across time and space. But if people understand themselves primarily as related social entities, then there is no universal person, female or otherwise. Rather each person is the composite of their social relationships. In other words, the rules that are part of the Safe Motherhood campaign forward a picture of social life that is utterly at odds with women, their family, and midwives' understandings of problems and risk. Problems and risk index, and emanate from, the birthing event itself. Problems are held to arise precisely because of the behaviors, beliefs, and practices of the particular people involved in the birth.

A more concrete illustration of the link between pregnancy or birth-related difficulties and the connectivity of the subjects can be found in the firestorm of blame that followed Rosario's death, as discussed in the prologue. Interestingly, Rosario's parents were furious with their son-in-law for their daughter's demise. They felt that their daughter was the victim of witchcraft perpetrated by one of his ex-lovers. But rather than hunt down and blame the scorned woman who cursed Rosario, they blamed her husband. Certainly, this attribution of blame only becomes logical when you consider husband and wife as relational, conjoined roles. In other words, the presence of a scorned women mars not only the husband, but disrupts the matrimony. In this light we can understand why the scorned woman targeted Rosario, rather than the person of her husband directly.

The formation of biosocial subjectivities is clearly illustrated by the importance of completing a homebirth "normally." Problems are frequently not recognized as such and seeming irregularities are later rewritten as individual variation, with the effect of promoting social integration among families. The relationality of subjects is so strongly produced and reinstantiated during the process of giving birth that to do otherwise—that is, identify a problem in the biological process—is tantamount to threatening social harmony. The inability of a woman to birth "normally" can index and create problems (most importantly) between a woman and her husband, or a couple and both sets of their parents.

Against this backdrop, the global campaign for Safe Motherhood and the Ministry of Health assumed and promoted an understanding of birth, and birthing-related problems, as primarily biological. They viewed an out-of-control physiology as a random, not conscious, and therefore blameless event. This perspective, perhaps unintentionally, excises pregnancy-related problems from the very matrix that make them interpretable. In doing so it forwards an understanding of place in the world that is discrete and unrelated to others. Women's bodies could be treated and their complications understood without reference to whether they were wives or mothers. Accordingly, medical interventions occurred in a way that could subtly redefine a woman and her family by weakening their connections.

Conclusion

PUTTING THE "MATERNAL" BACK IN MATERNAL MORTALITY

In 1985, Maine and Rosenfield asked a pivotal question: Where's the "maternal" in "maternal-child health"? Why were we only focused on mothers' capacity to improve or endanger their children's health, rather than on the health of mothers in their own right? This simple question transformed our approach to maternal health and created a space for the international community to try to decrease maternal mortality. Yet over two decades later, our progress toward that goal is debatable.

What can we learn about maternal mortality from focusing on what it means to be a mother, rather than by focusing on the biomedical causes of mortality? Before I started this study I suppose that I would have responded to the question of "what does 'mother' mean?" in a superficial way—to me, a mother was a female person who had and took care of children. But what I found in Sololá was that while children might be central to this basic meaning of mother, the meaning of *becoming a mother* and *being a mother* could reach far deeper into the family. Motherhood was essential to reproducing families, not only because of the bodily production of future generations, but because pregnancy and birth were primary sites for tying the fates of families together. Families in Sololá were not static units, they were made through everyday interactions. Pregnancy and birth were events that required the participation of the entire family and provided members an opportunity to solidify their relatedness.

One's understanding of one's place in the social world is co-produced (Lock 2001) by biological events like pregnancy and birth, resulting in what I call biosocial subjectivity. Exploring what it means to be a mother has helped me understand how subjectivities in Santa Cruz are intimately tied to meaning-making concerning biological processes. The understanding of self and kin that emerges through biological reproduction is one that emphasizes connectivity and mutual responsibility over independence and individuality. It takes a family to have a baby—while women may gestate, their husbands, fathers, mothers, and in-laws all play roles that are perceived as crucial to the well-being of future generations. Perhaps this case is made even stronger in the fabled *couvade*, a term that describes when fathers experience pregnancy-related symptoms and sometimes birth (Belaunde 2001). I also see this point being made in Vietnam, where the decision to abort a baby with a fetal anomaly is decided by entire families, instead of individual women (and their partners) (Gammeltoft 2007). Tine Gammeltoft (2007:60) explains that "within this political community, concern for others is expressed by overseeing and taking care of them, rather than by setting them free." Thus, the responsibility of such a weighty decision does not fall on a woman alone.

The emphasis on relational subjectivities also means that birthing difficulties are not suffered by women alone. In his study of "lay therapy management groups" John Janzen (1978) thoroughly detailed the role of kin groups in Zaire in helping to decide not only what was wrong with a family member, but what sort of treatment he or she should receive. Decades later and halfway around the world, his descriptions of negotiations were quite illustrative for helping me understand what I was seeing. Janzen's work, however, provided limited insight into how a connected sense of self actually extended the involvement of kin in a birthing-related problem; in Santa Cruz, a birthing-related problem could be just as keenly felt by all who were responsible and connected to a woman as by the woman herself. For example, in Rosario's case, while it was her body that manifested a problem, from the point of view of both her parents and the public who gossiped about her death the cause of the problem was her husband's infidelity that sparked his lover to curse his wife in childbirth. When the causes of biological pathologies are seen as social, everyone within a family unit can be affected equally.

Yet the interpretation of pregnancy-related problems within the Safe Motherhood campaign in Sololá was very different. Taking its cue from the international Safe Motherhood Initiative, the causes of pregnancy-related problems were decisively rooted in causes of mortality: eclampsia, hemorrhage, infection, obstructed birth, and unsafe abortion. From this logic stemmed the idea that the best intervention was one that targeted medical personnel in the hospital and improved their skills, since it was these medical personnel who would encounter the failing pregnant, or birthing bodies. The physiology that is used here to define birth is the physiology of one individual woman. This individual is assumed to be a discrete unit that can be analyzed and treated independently from her social relationships. A view of birthing-related problems that so heavily privileges individual biologies also forwards a certain understanding of selves as autonomous.

The Safe Motherhood campaign in Sololá assumed autonomous subjectivity and, therefore, interventions into the everyday actions surrounding pregnancy and birth promoted an understanding of the self as independent. The front line of Safe Motherhood was prenatal counseling where women were introduced to the "danger signs" of pregnancy. Theoretically, each woman who went to the health post for a prenatal exam received a short talk on the danger signs and a large card with a graphic for each sign to help her better remember the lesson. Again, the "danger signs" support the primacy of the physiological aspects of pregnancy and birth. On the flipside of the "danger signs" card were graphics to help a pregnant woman construct her own emergency plan. She was reminded to save her pocket money for emergency transport, find someone to watch her kids, and to discuss her plan with her friends and family. Obviously, for a married woman to take this advice to heart and act on it would be to supplant her own family. It would be to rearrange her own causal attributions—to believe that causing disharmony in the family would have no consequences to her birth. She would have to believe that pregnancy was limited to herself as a biological container, and that birth problems were random, physiological malfunctions that occurred due to events governed internally. In short, she would not only have to transform her own understanding of her biology, but her own understanding of herself.

The focus of the Safe Motherhood campaign on the biomedical management of birth in the hospital was equally consequential. If a woman did go to the hospital for an obstetric emergency she was processed through to the maternity ward where, regardless of whether or not she had given birth, her family would have to leave her. The campaign put little to no value on the importance of families birthing together. Rather, the emphasis of the campaign was on exporting individual women from the village to the hospital.

That an autonomous subject is the assumed recipient of health development interventions does not at all strike me as unusual. Policies are decided in western institutions and, as Suad Joseph (1996) contends, there are presently no other viable subjects available in western discourse. Yet while tailoring interventions to an autonomous subject at the international level may have been an oversight, this point was certainly not irrelevant in Guatemala. On the contrary, the autonomous subjectivity that was embedded in the interventions was appealing. The interventions were predicated on imaginary clients who took individual responsibility for themselves: they were educated to understand birthing problems, they had plans to address those problems, and they came to the hospital to seek help. This autonomous individual represented the type of modern,[1] educated citizen who could move forward to build a new, unified nation.

If we consider subjectivity as biosocial, it is really no surprise that health workers see health development that attempts to remake reproductive practices as an opportunity to modernize states. Heather Paxson (2004), for example, provides a vivid account of Greece, where birth rates are declining and abortion rates are incredibly high. Greek obstetricians and family planners encourage particular contraceptive practices, which they not only view as a more modern fertility control than abortion, but as building the State by increasing family size. Van Hollen (2003) shows how health workers in India insert IUDs into poor, post-partum clients in order to promote a modern nationhood. In this case, modernity is represented by limiting women's fertility rather than by increasing it.

When health workers become agents of development, they become the nodes through which "modernity" is spread, and accordingly through which a space, and its inhabitants, get "modernized." While the particular practices that are endorsed by health workers may change, as Van Hollen (2003:205) puts it, "the balance of moral power remains the same." In essence, health workers make choices for the poor and illiterate because these individuals don't know how to act "modernly." While these actions may be intended as helpful, and are certainly paternalistic, the unintended consequence is frequently that the poor and illiterate are driven away from the very sources of care that they need. This is certainly a problem.

But these abuses are not inevitable, just as moving birth from the home to the hospital is not necessarily inevitable. Rather, each is the result, at least in part, of programs and policies that are trying to change reproductive practices. It is obvious that the effects of Safe Motherhood have strayed far from the intended impacts. Nevertheless, the only conversations that seem to hold real currency are ones that address impacts in terms of reduced deaths. I would disagree that this is a situation where the ends justify the means—instead I would argue that a responsible approach to changing reproductive practices is one that seriously considers the effects of policies. While this doesn't preclude a global campaign to make pregnancy safer, it does dictate a fuller examination of the implementation of global policies. If the moral imperative of thinking through the wider implications of health development is not convincing enough, it is obvious that ignoring these implications is not a practical approach to improving health.

Global Maternal Mortality:
A Chance to Make a Difference

As I take stock of current maternal health policy, I appreciate that moving toward a continuum of mother-child health is certainly a much more comprehensive and inclusive strategy to reduce maternal mortality than anything we have tried before. Nevertheless, I am concerned that the basis of that policy continues to take for granted that gains can be made by exporting women from the systems of care that they chose. In Sololá, women and their families choose iyoma as trusted providers. No matter how much the health system is strengthened through a continuum-of-care approach, birthing women will continue to be isolated from those systems until those systems embrace the iyom. As health workers in the Safe Motherhood campaign in Sololá were so intent on showing, the iyom could be the bridge.

Yet, right now, it's hard to see how that option could appear on the table. The focus of maternal child health remains firmly trained on skilled providers. And within the focus of this discourse, iyoma have nothing to offer. Essentially, they are treated as similar to family members, as people who might be able to offer support and comfort, but who have no real "skill" and, following from that I would argue, no real value. The "traditional birth attendant" has been swept out of the picture as a new cadre of skilled midwives have been written in. But the two are not equivalent.

As the deadline for the Millennium Development Goals moves closer and closer and we continue to fall behind on our commitment to maternal health (World Bank and International Monetary Fund 2008), we find Safe Motherhood at a crossroads: on the one hand, there is a seriously felt need to revisit our inadequate attempts to make pregnancy safer that is symbolized by the sacking of the SMI; on the other hand, there is the clear message that "we know what works" (Campbell and Graham 2006). Certainly as Oona Campbell and Wendy Graham (2006) suggest, health systems need to be strengthened and to have a more flexible, holistic response to improve maternal and child health, but as this study shows us, strengthening the health system is not enough. We need to consider what it is that women want and start working with them.

Currently, advocating for a woman's choice to use an "unskilled" midwife and have a homebirth is not a tenable position within the movement to make pregnancy and birth safer. Yet, as scary as the prospect might seem to biomedical professionals, it should be! By denying a voice and a space to those who advocate for these types of homebirths, the very people that the international community needs to reach to make birth safer are marginalized. Their voices are muted and no possibility of dialogue exists. Providing women with the best care possible should not be equivalent to choosing that care for them. It should involve a strong measure of figuring out what they value and trying to improve that. Understanding maternal mortality is just as much about understanding what it means to be a mother as it is understanding why women die from obstetric causes. To be successful, then, our responses need to accommodate motherhood.

One premise of this book is that making progress in decreasing global maternal mortality necessitates decentering the explicit emphasis on "mortality" that currently dominates our understanding of pregnancy-related death. My research has highlighted the "maternal" over the "mortality" by asking what it means to be a mother in one location where the global campaign takes place. The social state of motherhood remains central to choices that women and their families make about obstetric care. It is fruitless to design interventions to quell a hemorrhaging uterus without first taking stock of how women and their families decide what they want and need to make birth safer. These perceptions are intimately tied to understandings and desires concerning motherhood. In short, asking what it means to be a mother is indispensable to expanding our understanding of pregnancy and birth outcomes in different places.

NOTES

Prologue

1. My husband, who is a biological anthropologist, was with me in the field during my first year of fieldwork.

Introduction

1. Robbie Davis-Floyd's (1992) seminal work on the ritual technologization of biomedical birth is iconic of a genre that traces how women who deliver their children in hospital are separated from their context and disciplined into passive roles. This separation and objectification is often reviled and feared, if not resisted (Martin 1992). Many studies have also documented biomedical health workers' abuses of poor women during labor and birth (Allen 2002; Rivkin-Fish 2005; Sargent and Bascope 1997). Health systems have also taken advantage of pregnancy as a point of contact with poor women to carry out paternalistic family planning agendas (Van Hollen 2003).

2. I examine the campaign to end maternal mortality as a more general example of "global health development." The campaign is global in that it intends the policies that it promotes to be uniformly applicable to all locales that experience high maternal mortality. The policy agendas of this global campaign, which I treat in depth in chapter 3, frequently become the de facto agenda for private funders and NGOs. Through these funding mechanisms (or independently), they then become the agenda of many countries' ministries of health. So regardless of how uniform or seamless the effort to end maternal mortality, its intents and effects are to standardize approaches to maternal health around the world.

3. Numerous scholars have critiqued the characterizations that I discuss here. Mike Featherstone, Scott Lash, and Roland Robertson's (1995) volume on *Global Modernities* speaks against the over-emphasis on homogenization, positing that homogenization and heterogenization need to be analyzed side by side as dominant tropes of our time. Jan

Nederveen Pieterse's (1995) discussion of "globalization as hybridization" critiques the tendency to make "localities" seem passive rather than active. Nina Glick Schiller, Ayse Caglar, and Thaddeus C. Guldbrandsen (2006) and Anne Waldrop (2004) show how these issues can be remedied by minimizing the artificial divide between global and local, and instead emphasizing their intersection, or the "glocal" (see Englund 2002 and Markowitz and Uriely 2002 for a critique of what is or is not accomplished by this position). Below, I argue that questioning the "hegemonic version" has been and should continue to be a central part of the anthropological project. My point in defining a "hegemonic version" is to clarify what I am writing against.

4. See also Lisa Handwerker (2002) and Siegrid Tautz, Albrecht Jahn, Imelda Molokomme, and Regina Görgen (2000:699).

5. For example, see Ara Wilson (1998) and Aihwa Ong (1987).

6. Don Kulick (1992) also illustrates this point in his monograph that counters the assumption that language loss is necessarily a product of globalization.

7. See also Applbaum (2000).

8. While I think that Blaney does a good job of characterizing why students might be challenged to be "humbled" without the help of a professor, I find that the division he sets up between student and teacher a bit objectionable. I perceive the disruption of the privilege encoded in a hegemonic global narrative as a conversation, among my students, myself, and a diverse body of scholars. Blaney's construction occludes that I myself might have anything to learn from this process. Our own social positions are under constant negotiation and redefinition as our relative power, ability, rank, gender, etc., changes. Understanding, then, what constitutes relative privilege is a constant process, not a finite one as Blaney implies. Nonetheless, his main point concerning how we teach to stimulate critical thought about one's own positional is well taken.

9. Over the last two decades a number of excellent anthropological works have helped us push further our understanding of bodies and embodiment as social phenomenon (see for example Turner 1995). Margaret Lock and Judith Farquhar's (2007) edited collection *Beyond the Body Proper* may be the most comprehensive attempt to synthesize different perspectives. By separating this work from my own, I do not mean to imply that bodies are always passive objects, as they both produce the social and stand as a product of it. Nevertheless, I concentrate more heavily on how everyday social actions produce internal understandings of one's place in the world vis-à-vis the body.

10. Anthropology as a discipline has produced a plethora of excellent work emphasizing the role of social processes in shaping subjectivities (Das 2000; Mahmood 2005; Biehl, Good, and Kleinman 2007), yet the relationship between biological processes and these social processes has been less directly interrogated.

11. Anthropologists have argued that relatedness can be established through everyday interactions as well as through blood and marriage. When I talk about defining kinship "processually" I mean that I focus on the actions and interactions that bind people together and build relationships of relatedness. What these particular actions might look like vary and have, for example, been described by Mary J. Weismantel (1995), Jessa Leinaweaver (2008), Isabella Lepri (2005) for indigenous South Americans, and Janet Carsten (1995) for Malaysians.

12. Strathern's (1988:6) work touches both on the constitution of persons and "human subjects." Anthropological works on personhood have certainly helped forged the argument that some people understand themselves more relationally than others (Mauss 1985; Schweder and Bourne 1984; Conklin and Morgan 1996). Yet, as illustrated by Jean and John Comaroff (2001), questions of person are interested in official and externally recognized social standing. While all people are subjects and all people have an understanding of their place in the world (subjectivity), not all subjects are persons. I part with discussions of personhood here. I am interested more in questions of subjectivity than person.

13. Maya Unnithan-Kumar (2004:5) invokes the term "collective ownership" to "refer ... to those instances where the *body* is primarily constituted through others" (emphasis added). She draws on this concept to examine how "techniques of assisted conception may not result in ... conferring an individual identity on the fetus, as they would in societies where bodies are considered to be individually owned." While there are certainly similarities between this analysis and my own, I invoke biosocial subjectivities to center us in internal processes of meaning-making.

14. Alternatively, discourses of birthing problems that finger the actions of loved-ones and relatives, such as having an affair or not loving enough, as criminally colluding to cause Rosario's death, reinstantiate and generate relational, connective subjectivities.

15. Ethnographically, Sherry B. Ortner (1989) and Aihwa Ong (1987) provide excellent examples of the latter.

16. Here I draw mainly on ethnographers of speech to make my point. For example, Don Kulick (1992) and Susan Gal (1979) have traced speech practices in multilingual communities to show how transitions from one language or register to another are intimately connected to speakers perceptions of questions of larger political-economy.

17. My theoretical framing of this topic has been heavily influenced by scholars who view language as social action, and track how meaning is derived through linguistic practices. This would include ethnographers of speaking, like Richard Bauman and Joel Sherzer (1974) and Dell Hymes (1973), and anthropologists who view language as social action (see for example Duranti 1994; Briggs 1992; Hanks 1990; Irvine 1989; Tedlock and Mannheim 1995; Reichard 1944).

18. The formal name of the Guatemalan Ministry of Health is El Ministerio de Salud Pública y Asistencia Social. This translates into English as the Ministry of Public Health and Social Assistance. I use the Spanish acronym MSPAS or the generic English shorthand of the Ministry of Health to refer to this agency.

19 In Kaqchikel, *"iyom"* is the singular of *"iyoma."*

20. Part of this mistaken assumption undoubtedly derived from the fact that my pilot study involved interactions between women in Ministry of Health posts and in out-patient care in the hospitals. In these venues women were not accompanied by other members of their family.

21. Though she had no problem with me using the recording for my study, she was too tired to participate in the interview. When I went back she had already gone home. I did, however, interview her family members when they brought her in.

Chapter 1

1. Purportedly, the village was originally located on the shores of the lake, but was wiped out by a landslide. The survivors then moved to the present location. Structures along the shore are certainly prone to be taken by landslides, swelling creeks that create rivers and lead to floods.

2. The word *muchacha* refers in Spanish to a young woman, and indeed, younger women normally fulfill these roles. Nevertheless, there is no age restriction concerning who can work as a muchacha.

3. The Kaqchikel term *mo's* is used locally to denote people who do not claim indigenous decent, and is the primary conceptual divider for identifying outsiders. Mo's applies equally to people from Guatemala City as it does to westerners of European decent. This may explain some of the flexibility in the deployment of words like *gringo*. While for many Latin Americans the term *gringo* is politically loaded, specifically divides people into US born and non-US born, and invokes resistance to imperialism, in Santa Cruz *gringo* is most frequently used as the Spanish equivalent of *mo's*. Under this system of classification Fidel Castro would be referenced as a gringo if he visited Santa Cruz. In this context gringo is not pejorative, and throughout this book I follow the locally prescribed norms for its use. (I thank Robert Hamrick for drawing this to my attention).

4. *Quetzal* (Q) is the currency in Guatemala. At the time of research the exchange was about 7.7 Q to $1 US.

5. In Guatemala the path to becoming a teacher involved six years of elementary, three years of general secondary education, then three more years of specialized secondary education, where students concentrated on teaching, business/accounting, or general baccalaureate. Completing the teaching degree necessitated only one more year of post-secondary

work. It was very difficult for people in Santa Cruz to complete all of this school, because it necessitated living outside of the village. While some schools were better at preparing teachers than others, frequently students received little training in pedagogy.

6. Two predominant alcohols were available in Santa Cruz, beer and *cux*, a high proof alcohol that was locally fermented. A fifth of cux costs about 1 Q, while a beer costs 5 to 7 Q. With a few fifths it was quite easy to get completely drunk.

7. There is some debate over how accurate his assertion was. Wenda Trevathan (1987), who provides references for this debate, discusses the evidence for and extent of giving solitary birth around the world, as well as arguing for the importance of a helper in the human evolution of birth.

8. Michele R. Rivkin-Fish (2005) discusses the slippage in assumptions that ties the veneration of choice in birth to feminism. Her reflections and analysis of conversations with a midwife working for the World Health Organization (WHO) about making birth in St. Petersburg more woman-centered are both riveting and enlightening.

9. Affines are in-laws.

10. A *t'uj* is a traditional sauna that most families have in their backyard. It is also referred to in Spanish as a *temascal*.

11. Interestingly, midwives also now receive cash from most families (many work on a "sliding scale" and only charge what they think someone's family can pay). Since how much a family has to pay is frequently a point of contention and gossip, I find it interesting that any reference to cash was omitted in my teacher's tale.

12. In their "three-delays" framework, S. Thaddeus and D. Maine (1994) identify the delay in diagnosing a problem as one of the major barriers to promulgating high rates of maternal mortality.

13. Lois Paul's (1975) protagonist, a midwife in San Pedro, was born with the same sign.

14. In the Mayan calendar, which dates from before the conquest, each day is named and traditionally children received their names for the day that they were born. Intertwined with your day and name is a particular destiny. The destiny describes your personal challenges and strengths and the certain roles that you can assume in society that will allow you to fulfill your life goals. While the Mayan calendar tells you who you will have to become to fulfill your destiny, it never assumes that you are bound to any one path. Nevertheless, it is difficult to walk down a path that is not yours, and sickness and bad events are predominantly interpreted as evidence that an individual is not following his or her destiny.

15. Cosminsky and Scrimshaw (1980) provide one of the most detailed accounts available of all of the different sources of power available to traditional healers.

16. The remaining two were charismatic Catholic, which meant that they attended the Catholic church when the priest would come, but built their own church that they attended more frequently, where they had prayer meetings and engaged in other activities (singing, for example) that the Evangelicals took for granted.

17. Cosminsky (2001:358) writes about the difference between a mother and daughter, who she has been following for almost forty years, and both of whom are midwives. Although the author does not comment on it, the daughter reports that one of the differences between her own practice and that of her mother is that she believes "only in God." Her mother, of course, drew on the help of a number of different spirits to do her work. This suggests that the erasure of spiritism from healing may be wider than just Santa Cruz.

18. A *corte* is a skirt that Mayan women traditionally wear.

19. My husband had returned to the hospital the same day we took Geronima in to help evacuate a man who had become intoxicated with a chemical and paralyzed. I stayed in the village the next day to make sure that his data collection kept going and he shuttled back to the hospital, talking to doctors and families of the two patients.

20. Later in the book I discuss in more depth the reasons why a family might not want to transfer a woman. Transferring patients like Geronima is very difficult for a family to bear because they do not have the resources to accompany their loved one. In short, families often prefer a less resourced hospital where a loved one can count on their own care, to a more technologically equipped hospital where they no longer can get any updates from their family member.

21. My perspective on how Geronima's case was handled in the hospital is very limited in comparison to other cases in this book because I had no direct access to either her chart or the medical personnel working with her. I would be quite surprised if the doctors on duty did not identify her eclampsia immediately, as pregnancy and convulsions are basically the tell-tale signs. What is most worrisome here is whether or not Geronima should have been transferred earlier. She was not conscious while I was with her and was convulsing regularly, suggesting severe pre-eclampsia or eclampsia. However, just because she was eclamptic did not mean that she would need to be immediately transferred. The ultimate treatment for severe pre-eclampsia or eclampsia is to deliver the baby, which happened about twenty minutes before arriving to the hospital. The protocol for treatment would then be to start a drip and administer magnesium sulphate and perhaps diazepam. Organ damage, particularly renal damage, is frequently the result of eclampsia, but there is no way that the doctors could have known the extent of the damage until some time passed. I can easily imagine a scenario where it takes far more than the three hours between when Geronima was dropped off and when her relatives would have to leave the hospital, to

get back the lab results showing whether or not her renal activity was improving or getting worse. Then everyone would have to wait until the morning to get the relatives' permission to move Geronima, as doctors can't make these decisions without the family's consent.

22. Though in the Spanish language there is technically no feminine form of *testigo*, *testiga* is used locally when referring to women.

23. In the one outlying case the midwife accompanied a woman with a retained placenta. Another unusual facet of this case is that she arrived carrying the baby. This is the only post-partum case that I recorded where the newborn was brought to the hospital.

24. M. Cameron Hay (1999) elucidates this point of view in her study of maternal death in Indonesia.

25. To put this act in context, health workers felt betrayed and despondent at Neli's action. They knew that she knew the guidelines, yet she chose to ignore them anyway. If she didn't follow biomedical protocol, they reasoned, who would? And if no one did, what would happen to the women who were dying the villages?

26. Sheila Cosminsky (1977a) also mentions this point. She relates that the Ministry of Health representative asked the midwives to bring all of their clients to the health center. When none showed, the representative asked why. The midwives said that the women didn't want to come. The representative said that they should have obligated them to. The midwives said that they didn't have the authority to do that.

27. Here I'm drawing on J. L. Austin's (1962) sense of how to do something.

28. Stack's (1974) groundbreaking ethnography does an excellent job of showing how important kin are to survival in low resource environments.

29. Kriemild Saunders (2002:21) offers a more comprehensive response to this sort of critique. She sees the value in the critique of a development project that I offer here as turning toward indigenous societies to offer "a valorization of modes of life devalued by modernity."

30. Not surprisingly, many anthropologists have demonstrated the propensity of development interventions to inevitably attempt to remake wider social life (see Ferguson 1990; Adams and Pigg 2005). Perhaps most relevant to my own work is Frederique Apffel-Marglin and Loyda Sanchez's (2002) work on state-sponsored reproductive programs in Bolivia. While the ostensible goal of the state was to promote contraception among poor indigenous women, Apffel-Marglin and Sanchez argue that the project encoded an ontology of being that envisioned women as discrete, human, and individual. This ontology, they argued, conflicted with indigenous ontologies (which emphasized continuity of beings), but was also instrumental in attempting to make individuated citizens for the Bolivian state.

31. Marcia Claire Inhorn (1996) traces two general understandings of patriarchy: a feminist one that is about oppression of women writ large

and a more anthropological one that defines patriarchy more literally—that is as the dominance of a patriarch or father of a family. My example tends to be more in line with the latter.

32. Interestingly, biomedical studies of the effects of labor support—that is allowing a woman to have a (female) companion with her during hospital labor and birth—began in Guatemala (Klaus et al. 1986; Sosa et al. 1980). The overwhelmingly positive effect of labor support on numerous measures relating to complications in labor and birth as well as outcomes for both mother and baby, led the authors to replicate the study in the US, where they found that the findings held (Kennell et al. 1991). Certainly the overall positive effect of having a caring companion in birth, and the lack of emphasis put on this factor in most hospitals, is also responsible for the increase in doulas in the developed world.

Chapter 2

1. In Chapter 3 I argue that the biologization and medicalization of birth is an inherent part of global Safe Motherhood efforts.
2. What is not represented in this transcript is the family's extensive conversations. Unfortunately, much of this talk took place directly outside of where the microphone was placed, and thus was not loud enough to hear.
3. Though I have never heard a story about the gate staff abusing a foreigner or a doctor, rumors abound about the gate staff refusing to let certain people in. A typical version of this story occurred right before I left the field. Apparently, the director of the hospital was entering the gate behind a patient and his family. The gatekeepers didn't see the director and began to harass the patient and refused to let him through. Witnessing the act of abuse, the director became irate. Families complain that they must spend twenty minutes in conversations with the gate keepers trying to get permission to pass. The gate keepers, of course, deny ever taking bribes or bothering patients and their families. Nevertheless, part of hospital reform in Sololá has been to emphasize that the role of the gate staff is to open and close the gate, not to decide who comes in and who doesn't.
4. Indeed, during my observation in the hospital I found that people did all three. During the day, however, there was typically a line of family members and people sitting on the benches waiting to get into the ER. If a patient was not at death's door, people usually just took a seat and waited for the door to open. If a patient's condition was grave, someone normally knocked on the door or walked into the ER itself. During my research I learned that the best way to arrive to the ER was with the firemen, who functioned as the ambulance service for the surrounding areas. The firemen would secure your direct passage into the ER itself without having to wait or knock, or negotiate the myriad people wait-

ing outside. They would also go and find the head nurse, which during the night, when s/he had ward duty as well as ER duties, was no simple feat.

5. In exit interviews with patients who were being discharged from the maternity ward, conducted by Jhpiego, participants overwhelmingly complained about the hospital gowns that they were forced to wear. Besides that fact that women don't like having to change, Sololá is cold, and the hospital, which is a cement block building, tends to get very chilly. The hospital gowns are like short nightgowns with cap sleeves—not much protection from the cold. A group of patients got together and designed an appropriate prototype for a gown, but since no funding was available to manufacture the garment, patients continued to be given the old, skimpy models.

6. This utterance is difficult to translate because the verb *quedarse* (to remain) is reflexive. Guadalupe's husband uses two different reflexive particles: "se," that would apply to a single person, and "nos," that applies to us. He is therefore being very vague and his question could be read to apply to how long Guadalupe has to stay in the hospital or how long her family will remain waiting for her.

7. After the family left the maternity ward, I interviewed them, and Guadalupe's husband said that he had not yet settled on a price for the trip with her uncle.

8. Again, she would be in no condition to travel on public transport.

9. It's unclear if the nurse knows exactly what is wrong with her immediately, as nowhere in the recording does the nurse ever ask why Guadalupe's family brought her. Nevertheless, she does know that this is an OB complication since she directs them to that part of the ER. She also can tell by Guadalupe's physique that she has recently given birth. This is probably sufficient information to surmise that her placenta is the problem. Regardless, parity itself is not going to be more important to a post-partum complication than, say, how long ago the baby was born, or when the complication started.

10. Again, this utterance is difficult to accurately translate because in English the verb "hurt" is the same in both present and past tense for third person plural, while in Spanish it is a different verb. In this utterance, the last time the nurse says "hurt," she says it in present tense.

11. I use "she" here referring to the midwife, but it is speculative. Guadalupe's husband uses the third person singular declination of the verb, but Spanish does not force him to either use a third person singular pronoun (e.g., he, she, or it) nor to gender the verb.

12. She was not communicative due to the Demerol.

13. Indeed, I observed other cases where swollen labia from repeated attempts to extract the placenta were an issue. In these cases, who had been trying to extract it was always an important question in the attempt to establish treatment history.

Chapter 3

1. In this chapter, I use "safe motherhood," without capitals, to refer to the general interest in reducing pregnancy-related death. When I capitalize "Safe Motherhood," I am explicitly referring to a program or initiative.

2. I have tried, as much as possible, to make this section as straight forward and reflective of what I consider the "timeline."

3. This focus on primary healthcare was the outcome of the International Conference on Primary Health Care that took place in Alma Ata, Kazakhstan, in 1978. At that meeting nations galvanized behind a broad definition of health and an approach to promoting health that went beyond the provision of institutional healthcare. Incorporating providers such as midwives was part and parcel of this approach and was, therefore, very popular. I discuss this point later in the chapter.

4. The term "traditional midwife" encompasses a particular world view that suggests a clean cut between "traditional" medicine and its supposed opposite, "modern" biomedicine. Margaret Jolly (2002) points out the incongruencies in this assumption. Marcia Inhorn (1994), among others, shows that midwives often are quite willing to learn or are even solicitous of biomedical practice to add to their repertoire. The term Traditional Birth Attendant (TBA) is also marked by a particular history more closely allied with the WHO, which I discuss below. I try to avoid both of these terms when referring to midwives with whom I had contact. However, in discussing literature and the opinions of others, I try to use the terms that individual authors or specific debates have employed.

5. Luc de Bern et al. (2003) theoretically ground the idea of "skilled attendance" and what it might mean. Martha Carlough and Maureen McCall (2005) provide an excellent overview of the concept and use the example of Nepal to show how it can be operationalized.

6. Obviously, not everyone would agree with this assessment. Oona Campbell and Wendy Graham (2006) argue that the evidence clearly points to the importance of the management of intrapartum care, and create an outline of an intervention based on that. A. Paxton et al. (2005) argue that emergency obstetric care does have the evidence base needed. Finally, Louise Ross, Padam Simkhada, and W. Cairns Smith (2005) argue that randomized control trials for maternal mortality interventions are just not practical, and thus, the idea of evidence based within this domain needs to be rethought.

7. Many estimate that of all the MDGs, the global community is currently most behind on improving maternal health (Rosenfield, Maine, and Freedman 2006).

8. There is no inherent conflict between these two paradigms—most agree on the benefit of merging them (Behague and Storeng 2008; Ooms et

al. 2008). Rifat Atun, Sara Bennet, and Antonio Duran (2008) add nu-
ance to these terms by dissecting the different levels at which programs
can be either vertical or integrated. While their approach suggests that
the divide is more rhetorical than actual, within the context of the Safe
Motherhood Initiative the division between vertical and horizontal has
been quite galvanizing.

9. While there is nothing wrong with prevention per se, it is more difficult to count cases prevented (because they never develop) than it is
to count lives saved through a curative intervention (like surgery). Understanding the outcomes of prevention strategies frequently occupies
a longer temporal space than measuring curative interventions.

10. Indeed, from the moment that comprehensive primary healthcare was
proposed, critics like Julia Walsh and Kenneth Warren (1980) have argued that the vertical disease control approach offers more bang for the
buck.

11. Technical strategies are, however, not as clean cut as many would
think. Jonathan Nathaniel Maupin (2008) describes some of the messi-
ness that is actually involved in extending midwife training as a line-
item for health system reform in Guatemala.

12. This included a form that was required to be filled out by an attending
physician for any pregnancy-related death in the hospital, a form that
had to be filled out by health workers in the village health posts and
health centers following any pregnancy-related death in a village and
finally, and in the absence of the first two, the investigation of every
death reported of a woman of reproductive age within Sololá to determine if her demise was pregnancy-related.

13. As this book goes to press, Margaret C. Hogan, et al (2010) argue that
rates of maternal mortality have actually decreased by 25% over the
last few decades. While these findings fly in the face of the estimates
of multilateral institutions, the authors argue that they have used far
more data points than competing reports. The editor of the journal *Lancet*, where the findings are published, claims that he was contacted by
maternal health advocacy groups asking to delay publication in the fear
that "good news" might decrease donor interest in funding maternal
health initiatives (Horton 2010).

14. Paul Farmer (1999; 2003) lays out an argument for how he sees health
as connected to human rights and why approaching human rights from
a health point of view (rather than, say, a traditionally legal one) might
be more effective. In writing about the relationship between neolib-
eralism, human rights, and reproductive health, Rosalind Petchesky
(2003) talks about the failure of market mechanisms to provide adequate health and healthcare, particularly in developing countries.

15. Ironically, the second legacy approach to maternal health, "Women
Deliver," is completely efficiency driven. The approach, which I discuss
in Chapter 5, seeks to convince that investing in women pays off in

terms of overall development outcomes. Many advocates were nervous about what Hogan et al's (2010) findings in the *Lancet* might do to the success of the second "Women Deliver" conference, which took place in the summer of 2010.

16. Guatemala is divided into "departments" rather than states or provinces.

17. This reflects a larger change in the official way to calculate the maternal mortality ratio, which went from deaths per any type of birth, to deaths per live births only.

18. I discuss the civil war in Guatemala more thoroughly later in the book.

19. I. B. Ahluwalia et al. (2003) describe a similar effort to develop emergency evacuation plans at the village level.

20. The yearly registers of maternal deaths in Sololá record the location of each death. In any given year there might be one or two hospital deaths, or even none. This seems counterintuitive, since one imagines the most at-risk population (that is, women with extreme complications) will be transported to the hospital. In actuality, though, many women die at home, or a few die on their way. Rosario's death, for instance, was recorded as having taken place in Santa Cruz, not in the hospital.

21. Midwives were not the only ones who were sensitive to the time scope of development programs. There seemed to be a general distrust of development projects because people were used to being abandoned. I saw the outcome of this in Tzununá, one of the villages where I worked: an entire complex of health buildings and a kindergarten were built and decorated, and enjoyed by the community for several years. They were then abandoned when the NGO that invested in the program failed to get follow-up funding. These buildings are now in disrepair.

22. Elena Hurtado (1984) provides a nice description of the "traditional" role of the sauna in homebirth in San Marcos. Notably, when I conducted interviews in San Marcos in 2002 and 2003 no one was using the sauna anymore. Also, the sauna was relied on more as a postpartum facility, rather than a place to give birth.

23. See Irene Figa'-Talamanca (1996) for a more successful description of how traditional midwives have been incorporated into a system of "waiting homes" in Columbia. A rural woman at risk can go to the waiting room and give birth with her midwife helping and present, in order to make sure that she is near more medical care should the need arise. I address what "real" integration in Sololá might look like in Berry (2005).

24. M. Catherine Maternowska (2006) provides an excellent description of how health workers can create and maintain a hierarchy within a clinic. Her example, which is from Haiti, illustrates the everyday means through which the work of those from the community can be denigrated by those with formal training.

25. In her book on post-Soviet reproductive health, Michele Rivkin-Fish (2005) provides one of the most in-depth discussions of tipping or bribing hospital workers, and the expectations of workers and clients surrounding these practices.
26. To put this into perspective, no nation on earth has registered a ratio that high.

Chapter 4

1. For a non-Guatemalan it will certainly be difficult to not be shocked by the apparent racist overtones in interactions like the one involving Petrona. Surely, race is prominent as an organizing feature of interaction in Guatemala. As one of Charles Hale's (2006:141) Ladino informants pointed out, "there is much discrimination against the indígena, so much that it has become part of Guatemalan culture."
2. Linda Green (1989) extends our understanding of the genuinely political nature of the national health system in Guatemala. During the early 1980s the Ministry of Health got on board the Health-for-All bandwagon and promoted primary healthcare as a model for addressing the health of its population. As Green argues, this primary healthcare model was particularly amenable to the State, since it did not ostensibly attempt to address the causes of poverties and inequities that underwrote the poor health of many disenfranchised and indigenous communities. But the broad constructions of health within the primary healthcare model lead primary healthcare workers to move beyond curative and preventative biomedicine, and to become community organizers and agitators. As a consequence the Ministry of Health pulled its support from primary healthcare and many of the primary healthcare workers were subsequently disappeared or assassinated by the military.
3. This situation was arguably not uncommon. During my research Jhpiego carried out a study of the time patients spent in outpatient care waiting to see a doctor versus the time they actually spent with the doctor. When the results were presented to the medical staff one patient had traveled two hours, waited an additional two and half hours, and was only seen for one minute. The doctors who staffed out-patient care were quick to explain this outlier by invoking the fact that patients frequently get referred to them when they should actually see another specialist.
4. This is a procedure where the uterus is physically scraped free of remaining material.
5. A *cuerda* is a unit of land like an acre.
6. Silvia was to live in a room that she shared with five other women. There is no public space or television in the hospital, so patients are essentially confined to their beds during their stay.

7. Unlike the other incidence of non-compliance that I witnessed, no one was outraged by Silvia's behavior; perhaps because everyone knew how absolutely difficult it was for her to comply with her doctor's medical recommendations. Later, one of the doctors drove to her house on a weekend to check up on her and to repossess the gown. Though Silvia's name never appeared on the department register for maternal mortality, I don't know what happened to her baby.
8. In Berry (2008) I discuss the issue of access to care and how many clients view health staff as gate keepers that restrict their access to cures.
9. A few minutes later two family members of another patient who were in the ER and listening to the conversation started joking with the doctor and the nurse about the man's stubbornness, making fun of him because he treated the staff as if they were the police and not healthcare professionals. Laughing, the doctor said, "We are obviously not the police, because the police will pry the truth out of you."
10. As Cosminsky and Scrimshaw (1980) point out, some healers made curative claims about the power of the IV.

Chapter 5

1. I am also upset that pointing out this prejudice alone is not seen as sufficient moral grounds for change, rather governments and donors must be convinced that allocating more money to women's health is an efficient investment.
2. The way that this argument that women are undervalued has been made is very similar to the logics that underwrote much of the theory of second-wave feminism. There is an assumption that one's status as a woman is her most important defining characteristic. Many women of color have productively rebutted this assumption by drawing attention to how class, racial, and ethnic identities frequently mean that they have more in common with men in their own groups than with any general category of women (Mohanty, Russo, and Torres 1991; Moraga and Anzaldúa 1983). Andrea Cornwall (2007) critiques the productivity of assumptions about mythical female unity within development.
3. This question has been answered in a number of ways. A dominant approach has been to focus on resources that poor people lack and how this impacts their obstetric care options. Poor people frequently do not live near biomedical care providers and they cannot pay to transport women in trouble nor for emergency or hospital care that they need (Renaudin et al. 2007; Thaddeus and Maine 1994). Another issue is that from a biomedical standpoint the care that poor people do receive from traditional providers in their homes is frequently judged to be substandard. Yet the poor frequently distrust the quality of the care that they will receive if they do go to a biomedical provider (Barnes-

Josiah, Myntti, and Augustin 1998; Berry 2008; Thaddeus and Maine 1994).

Another way to answer this question has been to unpack how biomedicine, as one way of knowing, can conflict with other ways of knowing that are prevalent around the world. For example, M. Cameron Hay (1999) argued that believing that fate dictates when one will die has stymied the efforts of the Indonesian government to increase skilled attendance at delivery. In this case women just do not agree that the biomedical proficiency of the birth attendant strongly determines the outcome of their birth. Rachel Chapman (2003) provides another provocative example of how women's beliefs in black magic trump any interest in seeking biomedical prenatal care. She reports how women view lining up at the clinic door as tantamount to admitting their early pregnancies, essentially announcing to their enemies that they are with a vulnerable, young fetus in their bellies. But sometimes the ideological conflicts occur within the biomedical providers themselves. Robbie Davis-Floyd (2003) theorizes that biomedical practitioners' rejections of traditional midwives and their knowledge can endanger the care a woman receives when transferred from a homebirth.

Yet another way the challenges of the everyday lives of the poor have been explored has been to consider how structural forces manifest and impact attempts to make pregnancy safer. For example, differences in ethnicity between provider and patient can complicate care-seeking behavior and the delivery of care (Glei and Goldman 2000; Glei, Goldman, and Rodriguez 2003; Maternowska 2006). To put it another way, women and their families may place more weight on who it is that will be attending them, rather than on their need for care, when deciding to seek biomedical attention or not. National policies both within and outside the realm of reproductive care can also arguably impact women's ability to access care (Janes and Chuluundorj 2004; Shiffman and Garcés del Valle 2006).

4. Linda Green (1994) describes the divisive impact of civil patrols where villagers informed on each other to the army. Civil patrols, however, were not universally exploitative, as Paul Kobrak (1997) so convincingly argues.

5. Patricia Lawrence (2000:177) discusses a similar situation in Sri Lanka, where the violence of the civil war created a situation where "the lines between who is friend and who is enemy have become impossible to draw."

6. There are several good historical accounts of the colonial period and Guatemalan history in general. Murdo MacLeod (1973) and Edwin Williamson (1992) provide good overviews that contextualize events in Guatemala and the larger colony.

7. Present day ladino identity is much more flexible, and describes anyone of any racial extraction that "exhibits the most important charac-

teristics of 'European' or 'national' culture, such as speaking Spanish or wearing non-Indian clothes" (McCreery 1994:9). The fluidity of these categories is also discussed by Kay B. Warren (1998), Carol A. Smith (1990a), and Charles R. Hale (2006). Neither Indian nor ladino identity is discrete or homogenous and individuals can move from one category to another.

8. David McCreery (1964) describes this system of labor recruitment and movement in detail.

9. Estimates of how many of Guatemala's 11,237,196 people (Instituto Nacional de Estadística 2002) are indigenous are difficult to come by since this is an inherently political question and ethnic categories are flexible. For example, are you indigenous if both of your parents are first-language K'iche' speakers, but you speak only Spanish and are a self-identified ladino? Early anthropology in Guatemala was particularly concerned with identifying ways to distinguish between indigenous groups and Antonio Goubaud Carrera (1964) summarizes and builds on these approaches. Nora England (2003), a scholar of Mayan languages, estimates that there are about thirty different Mayan languages spoken across Mexico, Belize, and Guatemala, while the Summer Institute of Linguistics (Gordon 2005), an evangelist group who acted as the government liaisons concerning indigenous languages throughout most of the last century, identifies fifty-four spoken dialects and two extinct languages in Guatemala alone.

10. With broad strokes, Jim Handy (1984) helps us understand much of the exploitation that has been the basis of state/indigenous relations even before ladino dominance of the country. Richard Newbold Adams (1970) presents a sobering account of state/indigenous relations over the mid twentieth century that highlights some of these shifts.

11. For a detailed account of the events that culminated in a vicious government anti-insurgency, see Gabriel Aguilera Peralta and John Beverly (1980). Robert Carmack (1988) provides an excellent description of this period.

12. Again, Green's (1989) detailed description of how healthcare workers could become targets of military violence helps us understand the extent of the threat felt by the State during this period.

13. Julie Hastings (2002), in writing about the paucity of first-person narratives concerning sexual violence during this period, gives us a sense of what sort of violence took place and why these narratives might be absent.

14. If upon entering a town all of the civilians had fled, the army would consider the inhabitants guilty and destroy the town anyway.

15. Smith (1990b) argues that eroding the autonomy of indigenous communities was a primary goal of the military during the civil war. When violence failed to do the job, they created model villages, where they forcibly resettled indigenous people. The purpose of this plan, Smith

reasons, was to use economic leverage to break community autonomy. Recent scholarship has critiqued the overly reified idea of autonomous Mayan communities inherited from Eric Wolf's (1957) work (Grandin 2000; Warren 2001). My analysis is not based on autonomy of communities writ large, but rather looks at individual actors within those communities and how they are coerced to participate.

16. In one instance, the perpetrator *was* a member of the security forces.

17. Indeed I never did.

18. San Pablo is the only village in the health district that boasted a health center rather than just a health post.

19. The popular sentiment that laws seem to protect criminals is applicable here. Godoy (1999) articulates this sentiment in relation to human rights. In a time of what is perceived as a crime epidemic, many Guatemalans see that human rights protocols only serve to protect the very criminals that prey upon them. Scheper-Hughes (1992) articulates the same argument for northeast Brazil.

20. In San Pablo an angry crowd beset a traveling group of HIV educators in the health center when one of the members was unduly rough with a child. In San Marcos villagers almost lynched the police for bashing in the head of a drunk man while trying to get his gold teeth so that they could sell them. In Santa Cruz villagers beset the office of the mayor, claiming that he was illiterate and incompetent. In San Pedro a teenager was lynched by his extended family for essentially being a rotten apple. I also followed several dramas that resulted in lynchings through the newspapers.

21. Travel by boat is relatively costly in comparison to bus. A twenty-minute boat trip into town is 4 Q, while a comparable bus ride is no more than 1.50 Q. The round trip to the Friday market in Sololá, the largest market for comestible goods in the area, is 11 Q (almost half a day's wage).

22. Only a few people in town owned refrigerators or freezers since they are expensive to buy and run. Lack of refrigeration eliminates the possibility of selling meat, and consequently, meat was only regularly available on Saturdays, when one woman sold fried chicken.

23. Though many say they end up breaking even or sometimes losing money growing their own corn, some families tend their own plots regardless of the costs. Sheldon Annis (1987) argues that the production of milpa, the plots where the corn is grown, is connected to organizing systems of belief.

24. I found that 40 and 50 year olds were the last generation for whom migration was common. While I was in Santa Cruz, a couple of young men went to try their hand at the coffee harvest, but when I asked about it most people said that the young men wanted to see what it was like to work outside of the village, take care of themselves, and meet other people.

25. Contractors in Santa Cruz pay workers less than the same daily wage as they would for equal work in Panajachel (a larger, more expensive town), but to work in Panajachel a man would have to either take a round-trip boat ride every day, or rent a room, both of which obliterate the profit differential.

26. The gringo/guardian relationship frequently mirrors the patronage bond established with godparents. Melvin Marvin Tumin (1952) provides a good description of the institution of godparents in Guatemala. He writes that indigenous Guatemalans frequently choose ladinos to be the godparents of their children, establishing this relationship so they have a wealthier or more powerful ally to call on in a time of need. Catherine Allen (1988) describes the same system in the Andes among Quechua and non-indigenous Peruvians. *Guardianes* frequently seek the help of their employers for favors and financial assistance.

27. "Benefits" in Guatemala generally mean that every June and December workers receive double salaries; thus, they earn fourteen months of salary over a twelve-month period. Permanent workers also receive what is called "*tiempo,*" i.e., they are legally paid one month of salary for every year they work in a location upon their expulsion or retirement from the job. This is supposed to provide a safety net for workers in a system where unemployment compensation from the government is not available. For some workers, benefits also include being included in the national social security system, which confers upon them rights to use the public social security health system (IGSS), supposedly a more endowed system than the general hospital system.

28. It should be noted that there is no minimum wage for agricultural workers or day laborers in Guatemala. Most Cruceños charged foreigners the same or marginally more for their labor as they did fellow villagers. How much one should pay laborers was a constant conversation among foreigners. Some felt that increasing salaries was important to increasing standards of living in the village. Others argued that increasing would just lead to more inflation in the village, making it harder for many to get by, and ultimately only benefitting the middle men.

29. Terracing is not practiced.

30. David McCreery (1994) argues that while many scholars have attempted to simplify tension over land in Guatemala as the result of the land grab that occurred during the initial development of the coffee plantations and the dispossession that followed, evidence of land disputes predates independence and has been just as prevalent between indigenous peoples themselves as well as between colonizers and indigenous. Greg Grandin's (2000) excellent account of class tensions between elite and peasant K'iche' tracks how peasants who used to farm communal lands become landless laborers for elite K'iche'. A similar transition has obviously happened in Santa Cruz.

31. In 2006, the first Cruceño finally found a way to the get to the US. Migration for young men, predominantly to Houston, has become possible.
32. Such stories are reminiscent of the *pishtacos* (mythical murderers) that Mary Weismantle (2001) writes about.
33. By my second year of fieldwork, I too became used to being hungry. Despite the fact that I spent almost every Friday morning going to the market and had no financial barriers to nutrition, I ended up losing eighteen pounds over the final twelve months I was in the field.
34. There are other important ways that the description of medicalization in Bom Jesus differs from that here. While the primary form of care for residents of the Alto was biomedical, that is not the situation with indigenous poor in Sololá. As I describe in the next chapter, Maya are very syncretic in their pursuit of a cure. At the hospital I saw patients fetishsize biomedical solutions (Berry 2008), but they do not venerate them as poor in Bom Jesus seem to.

Chapter 6

1. Talking about someone dying in birth was seen as bad luck, so many women just didn't want to engage the question, whether or not it was about themselves, someone they knew, or a hypothetical person.
2. One of the obligations that the government accepted in the Peace Accords was to extend medical services to the entire country. The training of midwives was included in these services. If there was no Ministry of Health presence, the government promised to contract a provider to visit the village and meet with midwives once a month. In the more distant aldeas of Santa Cruz this indeed happened. Maupin (2008) provides a detailed description of how this contracting worked in another Kaqchikel department.
3. Brigitte Jordan (1989) cites the importance of appropriate didactic methods and materials to teach Mayan midwives. The Ministry of Health obviously worked hard to produce appropriate materials that were picture-based rather than word-based and activities that were experiential rather than theoretical.
4. One of the dominant approaches to understand this phenomenon has been to try to see if midwives actually understand the materials (de León López 1987). Others, trying to put a more gentle spin on this same line of reasoning, say that the material is so complicated that it is unreasonable to expect most anyone to be able to apply it (de Bernis et al. 2003). Others have argued that the courses themselves are impoverished (Jordan 1989). Kruske and Barclay (2004), however, contend that the ways midwives are denigrated—like referring to them as "unskilled"—are typical of processes that do not seek to engage them as equals. Why should midwives cooperate in a process that does not

really include them as stakeholders? I also engage this question of what genuine participation of midwives in the health system must look like (Berry 2005). Kruske and Barclay's perspective certainly seems supported by the success that Johkio, Winter, and Cheng (2005) had in training midwives through participatory processes.

5. Margaret Jolly (2002) has asked us to question this neat divide between "modern" practices that are invasive and "traditional" practices that are more natural. She uses examples from Papua New Guinea (PNG) to show that "traditional" practices regarding pregnant and birthing women were often quite invasive, regulating even intimate practices like lactation and sex. "Modern" biomedical facilities in the outpost of PNG frequently lack the technology to be invasive. While there are undoubtedly differences between the ways that iyoma practice and the practices of the hospital in Sololá, as Jolly has demonstrated the use of "modern" and "traditional" tends to obscure, rather than elucidate, what they are. In this context, biomedical healthcare workers tended to use "traditional" to mean that the practices have not changed for millennia, and, therefore, were out of date. Quite the contrary, iyoma were very eclectic in their approach to managing pregnancy and birth, and were constantly incorporating new elements of practice, particularly biomedical ones (see Inhorn 1994 for a similar description of how "traditional" practitioners incorporate biomedical practices).

6. While this might not be a complicated problem for an obstetric specialist to resolve, the average doctor performing these surgeries was a general practitioner.

7. Men complained vociferously, since the health post was open only during the exact hours that they were working.

8. Many resented the amount of time the nurse spent vaccinating. International vaccination efforts were well funded and participation in the vaccination campaign was one of the main measures by which auxiliary health-post nurses' performances were evaluated. They were obligated to keep strict track of who needed to be vaccinated and to pursue those children in their homes. Many villagers didn't like having their children vaccinated because it gave them fevers. The Ministry of Health did not have enough acetaminophen to give to parents whose children were vaccinated, so frequently mothers would have to care for a sick child after the vaccination. I witnessed families hiding inside their houses, quietly waiting for the nurse—who was there to vaccinate—to go away. Invoking "the vaccinator" was also a popular measure to keep children in line. When I would visit people in their homes, mothers would tell misbehaving children that if they didn't shape up, I would vaccinate them.

9. A doctor and a professional nurse both staffed the health center, yet they were supposed to attend all 15,469 people who lived in the their health district.

10. While any sick person with an acute condition could be treated in the emergency room, the hospital also offered out-patient care, which functioned like a visit to the doctor. Patients arrived at the hospital from 7:00 AM onward and were given a number to see one of four medical specialists or the dentist. The consultation was free, but patients had to purchase any prescriptions. Medicines were available at discount prices from the hospital's own pharmacy. People in Santa Cruz used the hospital frequently for things such as getting stitches, pulling teeth, obtaining an ultrasound or an X-ray, and visiting other patients.

11. In her thesis, Caroline Rosenthal (1987) documents the reliance of villagers on the pharmacist for treating them and prescribing drugs.

12. Many anthropologists have made the same argument. Many essays from both Jolly's (2002) and Robbie Davis-Floyd and Carolyn Sargent's (1997) volumes challenge the idea that biomedicine is a monolithic entity, especially in relation to birth.

13. The central importance of trust in dictating which healthcare provider an iyoma recommended turning to was illustrated over and over during my fieldwork. Amalia's story of arriving to the hospital accompanying a client who she thought was carrying twins is typical. One baby had been birthed quite easily, but Amalia still felt another baby high up in her client's uterus. When it didn't come out they called a private doctor who told them that the woman would have to go to the hospital and have a c-section to deliver the second twin. The midwife told the family to find transport and then she led them to the hospital in Sololá. Though this family was from Tecpán, a relatively large city twenty kilometers away on straight roads from the hospital in Chimaltenango, the midwife said it was better to go to Sololá, which was sixty kilometers away, separated from Tecpán by a windy mountain road and more expensive to reach. She told me that she preferred Sololá because they always attended emergencies directly and, most importantly for her, they always let her stay with her clients. She said that the staff in the Sololá hospital had respect for midwives and treated her well. She would, therefore, always work with Sololá hospital when given a choice.

14. In Berry (2005) I provide a more detailed illustration of how iyoma find guidelines inappropriate for their practices, which are heavily predicated on tailoring to the characteristics of each individual woman. In this instance, iyoma could not agree with health workers that one can set a time after which you know a baby will not change position in utero.

15. Chapman (2003; 2006) also finds a strong link between witchcraft and perceptions of pregnancy-related problems.

16. Denise Roth Allen (2002) reports a similar interpretation of birthing difficulties in Tanzania, where a woman with problems in her birth was forced to "confess" a seemingly non-existent affair. This clandestine affair was perceived by the attendant to be the root cause of her problems.

17. Margaret Lock and Patricia Kaufert's (1998) volume also speaks to women's own practicality and agency in their choice-making surrounding reproductive issues. Carla Obermeryer (2000) demonstrates the same point through an examination of Moroccan women's choices about pregnancy-related care.

18. While our understanding of how different parties calculate risk has been significantly enriched by the works of psychologists Amos Tversky and Daniel Kahneman (Tversky and Kahneman 1973, 1974, 1986; Kahneman and Tversky 1972), anthropologists have also been prolific in writing about differing notions of risk. Many of the essays in Barbara Harthorn and Laury Oaks's (2003) edited volume help us understand how political, economic, and social trends can shape our understanding of dangers associated with a particular health issue. Hay (1999), Allen (2002), and Chapman (2003) all discuss differing perceptions of risk within the context of health programs to make pregnancy and birth safer.

19. I explain these concerns more thoroughly in Berry (2008).

20. This example is admittedly reactionary and is not meant to be any reflection on Afghan hospitals. I think that what worked about this example was not the fact that anyone I was talking to, including myself, knew anything about Afghan hospitals, but rather that we were in a state of war, and using the example of falling behind enemy lines was somehow intuitively accessible.

21. Obviously, autopsies are not procedures that have any therapeutic benefits. I only mention them here because many women were transported to the hospital with an obstetric emergency only to arrive dead (like Rosario). These women were required to have an autopsy. According to Guatemalan law, all individuals who do not die of known causes in front of an official (judge, policeman, fireman, doctor, etc.) must undergo an autopsy to determine the cause of death. One the one hand, it is obvious how important this law could be to preventing murder. However, it ignores the fact that most (particularly poor) indigenous people were opposed to the system of autopsies. In general, this was not a difficult position to understand in Santa Cruz where all-night wakes were open casket and no morticians were available to erase the marks of the pathologist's scalpel.

22. A number of authors have written about the connection between blood donation and nationalism. See Cohen (2001), Seeman (1999), and Simpson (2009).

23. Technically, pastors allied themselves with existing Evangelical denominations. When I asked congregants what this meant they told me that they paid fees to their headquarters in Sololá, and that their denomination determined a particular friend network for them. For example, youth from one church in Santa Cruz might meet with members of a church of the same name in Panajachel.

24. In contrast, while the Catholic laity might apply the idea of sins that they learned at church to judge themselves and others, the Church writ large was uninvolved in publicly managing the lives of the parishioners. The Catholic sermons had nothing to do with local circumstances and one member's transgressions were certainly not a possible topic, as much because the priest had no idea what was going on in individuals' lives as this would be inappropriate. Parishioners learned lessons about being Catholic but it was up to them to figure out how to apply these lessons.

25. The punitive stance toward alcohol consumption in the evangelical church was reason enough for many women to join and practice. The evangelical orientation toward social control and penalties for transgressing religious edicts was attractive to many women who lacked the power in their own lives to counter their husbands. It was both safer and more forceful to tell your husband, "God does not want you to drink and God will punish you for your transgression," than to say, "I want you to stop drinking."

26. This position is not as unusual as it might seem. The highest recorded rates of maternal mortality for any one group in the world occurred among the Faith Assembly in Indiana, where women birthed at home with family members for religious reasons (Spence, Danielson, and Kaunitz 1984; Kaunitz, Spence, and Danielson 1984).

27. When I later asked Sofia she told me that she did not have any such conversation with Ofelia.

Conclusion

1. Again I am referring to Jameson's (2002) understanding of the term as I discussed in chapter 4.

BIBLIOGRAPHY

AbouZahr, Carla. 2003. "Safe Motherhood: A Brief History of the Global Movement 1947–2002." *British Medical Bulletin* 67:13–25.

AbouZahr, Carla., and Tessa Wardlaw. 2001. "Maternal Mortality at the End of a Decade: Signs of Progress?" *Bulletin of the World Health Organization* 79 (6):561–68.

Abu-Lughod, Lila. 1990. "The Romance of Resistance: Tracing Transformations of Power Through Bedouin Women." *American Ethnologist* 17 (1):41–55.

Adams, Richard Newbold. 1970. *Crucifixion by Power; Essays on Guatemalan National Social Structure, 1944–1966.* Austin: University of Texas Press.

Adams, Vincanne, and Stacy Leigh Pigg. 2005. *Sex in Development: Science, Sexuality, and Morality in Global Perspective.* Durham: Duke University Press.

Agrawal, Arun. 2005. *Environmentality: Technologies of Government and the Making of Subjects, New Ecologies for the Twenty-First Century.* Durham: Duke University Press.

Ahluwalia, Indu. B., et al. 2003. "An Evaluation of a Community-Based Approach to Safe Motherhood in Northwestern Tanzania." *International Journal of Gynecology & Obstetrics* 82 (2):231–40.

Allen, Catherine J. 1988. *The Hold Life Has: Coca and Cultural Identity in an Andean Community.* Washington, D.C.: Smithsonian Institute Press.

Allen, Denise Roth. 2002. *Managing Motherhood, Managing Risk: Fertility and Danger in West Central Tanzania.* Ann Arbor: University of Michigan Press.

Amnesty International. 2005. *Guatemala: No Protection, No Justice: Killings of Women in Guatemala.* London: Amnesty International.

———. 2006. *Guatemala: No Protection, No Justice: Killings of Women in Guatemala* (an update). London: Amnesty International.

Annis, Sheldon. 1987. *God and Production in a Guatemalan Town.* Austin: University of Texas Press.

Apffel-Marglin, Frederique, and Loyda Sanchez. 2002. "Developmentalist Feminism and Neocolonialism in Andean Communities." In *Feminist Post-Development Thought: Rethinking Modernity, Postcolonialism and Representation,* ed. K. Saunders. London: Zed Books.

Appadurai, Arjun. 1990. "Disjunctures in the Global Cultural Economy." *Theory, Culture and Society* 7:295–310.

Applbaum, Kalman. 2000. "Crossing Borders: Globalization as Myth and Charter in American Transnational Consumer Marketing." *American Ethnologist* 27 (2):257–282.

Asowa-Omorodion, Francisca Isibhakhome. 1997. "Women's Perceptions of the Complications of Pregnancy and Childbirth in Two Esan Communities, Edo State, Nigeria." *Social Science & Medicine* 44 (12):1817–1824.

Atun, Rifat A., Sara Bennett, and Antonio Duran. 2008. *When do Vertical (Stand-Alone) Programmes have a Place in Health Systems?* Copenhagen, Denmark: Regional Office for Europe of the World Health Organization.

Austin, John L. 1962. *How to Do Things with Words. The William James Lectures 1955.* Cambridge: Harvard University Press.

Bakhtin, Mikhail. 1981. *The Dialogic Imagination.* Austin: University of Texas Press.

Barnes-Josiah, Debora, Cynthia Myntti, and Antoine Augustin. 1998. "The 'Three Delays' as a Framework for Examining Maternal Mortality in Haiti." *Social Science & Medicine* 46 (8):981–993.

Bastien, Joseph W. 1985. "Qollahuaya-Andean Body Concepts: A Topographical-Hydraulic Model of Physiology." *American Anthropologist* 87 (3): 595–611.

Bauman, Richard, and Joel Sherzer. 1974. *Explorations in the Ethnography of Speaking.* London, New York: Cambridge University Press.

Behague, Dominique. P., and Katerini T. Storeng. 2008. "Collapsing the Vertical-Horizontal Divide: An Ethnographic Study of Evidence-Based Policymaking in Maternal Health." *American Journal of Public Health* 98 (4):644–649.

Belaunde, Luisa Elvira. 2001. "Menstruation, Birth Observances and the Couple's Love Among the Airo-Pai of Amazonian Peru." In *Managing Reproductive Life: Cross-Cultural Themes in Sexuality and Fertility,* ed. S. Tremayne. New York: Berghahn Books.

Bernstein, Basil. 1975. *Class, Codes and Control: Theoretical Studies towards a Sociology of Language.* New York: Shocken.

Berry, Nicole S. 2005. "Incorporating Cultural Diversity into Health Systems: An Example of Midwives Teaching Midwives." *Women in International Development Forum* XXVII (January):1–9.

———. 2008. "Who's Judging the Quality of Care? Indigenous Maya and the Problem of 'Not Being Attended.'" *Medical Anthropology* 27 (2):164–189.

Biehl, João Guilherme, Byron Good, and Arthur Kleinman. 2007. *Subjectivity: Ethnographic Investigations, Ethnographic Studies in Subjectivity.* Berkeley: University of California Press.

Blaney, David L. 2002. Global Education, "Disempowerment, and Curricula for a World Politics." *Journal of Studies in International Education* 6 (3): 268–282.

Bledsoe, Caroline H. 2002. *Contingent Lives: Fertility, Time and Aging in West Africa.* Chicago: University of Chicago Press.

Boddy, Janice Patricia. 1989. *Wombs and Alien Spirits: Women, Men, and the Zar Cult in Northern Sudan, New Directions in Anthropological Writing*. Madison: University of Wisconsin Press.

Bogin, Barry, and James Loucky. 1997. "Plasticity, Political Economy, and Physical Growth Status of Guatemala Maya Children Living in the United States." *American Journal of Physical Anthropology* 102 (1):17–32.

Bourdieu, Pierre. 1991. *Language and Symbolic Power*. Cambridge, MA: Harvard University Press.

Briggs, Charles L. 2004. "Theorizing Modernity Conspiratorially: Science, Scale, and the Political Economy of Public Discourse in Explanations of a Cholera Epidemic." *American Ethnologist* 31 (2):164–187.

Briggs, Charles L., and Richard Baumen. 1992. "Genre, Intertextuality, and Social Power." *Journal of Linguistic Anthropology* 2:131–172.

Brotherton, P. Sean. 2008. "'We Have to Think Like Capitalists but Continue Being Socialists': Medicalized Subjectivities, Emergent Capital, and Socialist Entrepreneurs in Post-Soviet Cuba." *American Ethnologist* 35 (2): 259–274.

Brown, Penelope, and Stephen C. Levinson. 1987. *Politeness: Some Universals in Language Usage, Studies in Interactional Sociolinguistics*. Cambridge: Cambridge University Press.

Bullough, Colin et al. 2005. "Current Strategies for the Reduction of Maternal Mortality." *BJOG: An International Journal of Obstetrics and Gynaecology* 112 (9):1180–1188.

Campbell, Oona M. R., and Wendy J Graham. 2006. "Strategies for Reducing Maternal Mortality: Getting on With What Works." *Lancet* 368 (9543): 1284–1299.

Carlough, Martha, and Maureen McCall. 2005. "Skilled Birth Attendance: What Does it Mean and How Can it be Measured? A Clinical Skills Assessment of Maternal and Child Health Workers in Nepal." *International Journal of Gynecology & Obstetrics* 89 (2):200–208.

Carmack, Robert S. 1988. *Harvest of Violence: The Maya Indians and the Guatemalan Crisis*. Norman: University of Oklahoma Press.

Carsten, Janet. 1995. "The Substance of Kinship and the Heat of the Hearth—Feeding, Personhood, and Relatedness Among Malays in Pulau-Langkawi." *American Ethnologist* 22 (2):223–241.

Chapman, Rachel R. 2003. "Endangering Safe Motherhood in Mozambique: Prenatal Care as Pregnancy Risk." *Social Science & Medicine* 57:355–374.

———. 2006. "Chikotsa—Secrets, Silence, and Hiding: Social Risk and Reproductive Vulnerability in Central Mozambique." *Medical Anthropology Quarterly* 20 (4):487–515.

Cohen, Lawrence. 2001. "The Other Kidney: Biopolitics Beyond Recognition." *Body & Society* 7 (2–3):9–29.

———. 2003. "Where it Hurts: Indian Material for an Ethics of Organ Transplantation." *Zygon* 38 (3):663–688.

Comaroff, Jean L., and John Comaroff. 2001. "On Personhood: An Anthropological Perspective from Africa." *Social Identities* 7 (2):267–283.

Comisión para el Esclarecimiento Histórico (CEH). 1999. *Guatemala: Memory of Silence, Report of the Commission for Historical Clarification: Conclusions and Recommendations.* Guatemalan Historical Clarification Commission.

Conklin, Beth A., and Lynn M. Morgan. 1996. "Babies, Bodies, and the Production of Personhood in North America and a Native Amazonian Society." *Ethos* 24 (4):657–694.

Cooper, Frederick. 1994. "Conflict and Connection: Rethinking Colonial African History." *The American Historical Review* 99 (5):1516–1545.

———. 2001. "What is the Concept of Globalization Good for? An African Historian's Perspective." *African Affairs* 100 (399):189–213.

Cornwall, Andrea. 2007. "Myths to Live By? Female Solidarity and Female Autonomy Reconsidered." *Development and Change* 38 (1):149–168.

Cosminsky, Sheila. 1977. "Childbirth and Midwifery on a Guatemalan Finca." *Medical Anthropology* 6 (3):69–104.

———. 1977. "El Papel de la Comadrona en Mesoamerica." *America Indigena* 37 (2):305–335.

———. 1982. "Childbirth and Change: A Guatemalan Study." In *Ethnography of Fertility and Birth,* ed. C. P. MacCormack. London, New York: Academic Press.

———. 2001. "Midwifery Across the Generations: A Modernizing Midwife in Guatemala." *Medical Anthropology* 20 (4):345–378.

Cosminsky, Sheila, and Mary Scrimshaw. 1980. "Medical Pluralism on a Guatemalan Plantation." *Social Science & Medicine Part B—Medical Anthropology* 14 (4B):267–278.

Costello, Anthony, Kishwar Azad, and Sarah Barnett. 2006. "An Alternative Strategy to Reduce Maternal Mortality." *Lancet* 368 (9546):1477–1479.

Daniel, Valentine E. 1996. *Charred Lullabies: Chapters in an Anthropography of Violence.* Princeton: Princeton University Press.

Das, Veena. 2000. *Violence and Subjectivity.* Berkeley: University of California Press.

Davis-Floyd, Robbie. 1992. *Birth as an American Rite of Passage, Comparative Studies of Health Systems and Medical Care.* Berkeley: University of California Press.

———. 2003. "Home-Birth Emergencies in the US and Mexico: The Trouble with Transport." *Social Science & Medicine* 56 (9):1911–1931.

Davis-Floyd, Robbie, and Carolyn Fishel Sargent. 1997. *Childbirth and Authoritative Knowledge: Cross-Cultural Perspectives.* Berkeley: University of California Press.

de Bernis, Luc et al. 2003. "Skilled Attendants for Pregnancy, Childbirth and Postnatal Care." *British Medical Bulletin* 67 (1):39–57.

Delaney, Carol Lowery. 1991. *The Seed and the Soil: Gender and Cosmology in Turkish Village Society, Comparative Studies on Muslim Societies.* Berkeley: University of California Press.

de León López, Zoila Iris. 1987. *Evaluación de la Metodología Empleada en los Cursos de Adiestramiento a Comadronas Tradicionales en el Distrito de Salud de Mazatenango, Suchitepequez.* Facultad de Humanidades, Universidad de San Carlos de Guatemala, Guatemala.

Deneux-Tharaux, Catherine et al. 2005. "Underreporting of Pregnancy-Related Mortality in the United States and Europe." *Obstetrics & Gynecology* 106 (4):684–692.

Donnay, France. 2000. "Maternal Survival in Developing Countries: What Has Been Done, What Can Be Achieved in the Next Decade." *International Journal of Gynecology & Obstetrics* 70 (1):89–97.

Drew, Paul, and John Heritage. 1992. "Analyzing Talk at Work: An Introduction." In *Talk at Work: Interaction in Institutional Settings*, ed. Drew Heritage. Cambridge: Cambridge University Press.

Duranti, Alessandro. 1994. *From Grammar to Politics: Linguistic Anthropology in a Western Samoan Village.* Berkley: University of California Press.

England, Nora C. 2003. "Mayan Language Revival and Revitalization Politics: Linguists and Linguistic Ideologies." *American Anthropologist* 105 (4): 733–743.

Englund, Harri. 2002. "Ethnography after Globalism: Migration and Emplacement in Malawi." *American Ethnologist* 29 (2):261–286.

Farmer, Paul. 1992. *AIDS and Accusation: Haiti and the Geography of Blame, Comparative Studies of Health Systems and Medical Care.* Berkeley: University of California Press.

———. 1999. "Pathologies of Power: Rethinking Health and Human Rights." *American Journal of Public Health* 89 (10):1486–1496.

———. 2003. *Pathologies of Power: Health, Human Rights, and the New War on the Poor, California Series in Public Anthropology.* Berkeley: University of California Press.

Fauveau, Vincent, and France Donnay. 2006. "Can the Process Indicators for Emergency Obstetric Care Assess the Progress of Maternal Mortality Reduction Programs? An Examination of UNFPA Projects 2000–2004." *International Journal of Gynecology & Obstetrics* 93 (3):308–316.

Featherstone, Mike, Scott Lash, and Roland Robertson. 1995. *Global Modernities.* London, Thousand Oaks, CA: Sage.

Ferguson, James. 1990. *The Anti-Politics Machine: "Development," Depoliticization, and Bureaucratic Power in Lesotho.* Cambridge, New York: Cambridge University Press.

Figa'-Talamanca, Irene. 1996. "Maternal Mortality and the Problem of Accessibility to Obstetric Care: The Strategy of Maternity Waiting Homes." *Social Science and Medicine* 42 (10):1381–1390.

Forster, Cindy. 1999. "Violent and Violated Women: Justice and Gender in Rural Guatemala, 1936–1956." *Journal of Women's History* 11 (3):55–77.

Fortney, Judith A. 2001. "Emergency Obstetric Care: The Keystone in the Arch of Safe Motherhood." *International Journal of Gynecology & Obstetrics* 74 (2):95–97.

Foucault, Michel. 1973. *The Birth of the Clinic: An Archaeology of Medical Perception.* New York: Pantheon Books.

————. 1978. *The History of Sexuality.* 3 vols. New York: Pantheon Books.

————. 1983. "The Subject and Power." In *Michel Foucault, Beyond Structuralism and Hermeneutics,* ed. H. L. Dreyfus, P. Rabinow, and M. Foucault. Chicago: University of Chicago Press.

Freedman, Lynn P. et al. 2007. "Practical Lessons from Global Safe Motherhood Initiatives: Time for a New Focus on Implementation." *Lancet* 370 (9595):1383–1391.

Freire, Paulo. 1970. *Pedagogy of the Oppressed.* New York: Herder and Herder.

Gal, Susan. 1979. *Language Shift: Social Determinants of Linguistic Change in Bilingual Austria.* New York: Academic Press.

Gammeltoft, Tine M. 2007. "Prenatal Diagnosis in Postwar Vietnam: Power, Subjectivity, and Citizenship." *American Anthropologist* 109 (1):153–163.

Garrard-Burnett, Virginia. 2008. "Priests, Preachers, and Politics: The Region's New Religious Landscape." *Current History* 107 (February):84–89.

Geertz, Clifford. 1973. "Thick Description: Toward an Interpretive Theory of Culture." In *The Interpretation of Cultures: Selected Essays.* New York: Basic Books.

Gill, Kirrin, Rohini Pande, and Anju Malhotra. 2007. "Women Deliver for Development." *Lancet* 370 (9595):1347–1357.

————. 2007. "Women Deliver for Development: Background Paper for the Women Deliver Conference, 18–20 October 2007." Washington, DC: Family Care International and International Center For Research On Women.

Gish, Oscar. 1982. "Selective Primary Health Care: Old Wine in New Bottles." *Social Science and Medicine* 16 (10):1049–1063.

Glei, Dana A., and Noreen Goldman. 2000. "Understanding Ethnic Variation in Pregnancy-Related Care in Rural Guatemala." *Ethnicity & Health* 5 (1):5–22.

Glei, Dana A., Noreen Goldman, and German Rodriguez. 2003. "Utilization of Care during Pregnancy in Rural Guatemala: Does Obstetrical Need Matter?" *Social Science & Medicine* 57 (12):2447–2463.

Godoy, Angelina Snodgrass. 2000. "'Our right is the right to be killed': Making Rights Real on the Streets of Guatemala City." *Childhood* 6 (4):423–442.

————. 2002. "Lynchings and the Democratization of Terror in Postwar Guatemala: Implications for Human Rights." *Human Rights Quarterly* 24 (3):640–661.

Goldin, Liliana R. 2001. "Maquila Age Maya: Changing Households and Communities of the Central Highlands of Guatemala." *Journal of Latin American Anthropology* 6 (1):30–57.

Goldstein, Donna M. 2003. *Laughter Out of Place: Race, Class, Violence, and Sexuality in a Rio Shantytown.* Berkeley: University of California Press.

Gordon, Raymond G., Jr., ed. 2005. *Ethnologue: Languages of the World.* 15th edition. Dallas: SIL International.

Goubaud Carrera, Antonio. 1964. *Indigenismo en Guatemala, Publicación (Seminario de Integración Social Guatemalteca); no. 14.* Guatemala: Centro Editorial "José de Pineda Ibarra" Ministerio de Educación Pública.

Graham, Wendy J. 2002. "Now or Never: The Case for Measuring Maternal Mortality." *Lancet* 359:701–704.

Graham, Wendy. J., et al. 2008. "Measuring Maternal Mortality: An Overview of Opportunities and Options for Developing Countries." *BMC Medicine* 6 (1):12.

Graham, Wendy J., William Brass, and Robert W. Snow. 1989. "Estimating Maternal Mortality: The Sisterhood Method." *Studies in Family Planning* 20 (3):125–135.

Grandin, Greg. 2000. *The Blood of Guatemala: A History of Race and Nation.* Durham: Duke University Press.

Green, Lawrence W. 2006. "Public Health Asks of Systems Science: To Advance Our Evidence-Based Practice, Can You Help Us Get More Practice-Based Evidence?" *American Journal of Public Health* 96 (3):406–409.

Green, Linda. 1989. "Consensus and Coercion: Primary Health Care and the Guatemalan State." *Medical Anthropology Quarterly* 3 (3):246–257.

———. 1994. "Fear as a Way of Life." *Cultural Anthropology* 9 (2):227–56.

Hale, Charles R. 2006. *Más que un Indio: Racial Ambivalence and Neoliberal Multiculturalism in Guatemala.* Santa Fe. NM: School of American Research Press.

Handwerker, Lisa. 2002. "The Politics of Making Modern Babies in China: Reproductive Technologies and the 'New' Eugenics." In *Infertility Around the Globe: New Thinking on Childlessness, Gender, and Reproductive Technologies,* ed. M. C. Inhorn and F. van Balen. Berkeley: University of California Press.

Handy, Jim. 1984. *Gift of the Devil: A History of Guatemala.* Toronto: Between The Lines.

Hanks, William F. 1990. *Referential Practice: Language and Lived Space Among the Maya.* Chicago: University of Chicago Press.

Harthorn, Barbara Herr, and Laury Oaks, eds. 2003. *Risk, Culture, and Health Inequality Shifting Perceptions of Danger and Blame.* Westport, CT: Praeger.

Hastings, Julie A. 2002. "Silencing State-Sponsored Rape: In and Beyond a Transnational Guatemalan Community." *Violence Against Women* 8 (10): 1153–1181.

Hay, M. Cameron. 1999. "Dying Mothers: Maternal Mortality in Rural Indonesia." *Medical Anthropology* 18:243–279.

Hill, Kenneth et al. 2007. "Estimates of Maternal Mortality Worldwide Between 1990 and 2005: An Assessment of Available Data." *Lancet* 370 (9595):1311–1319.

Hinojosa, Servando Z. 2004. "Authorizing Tradition: Vectors of Contention in Highland Maya Midwifery." *Social Science & Medicine* 59 (3):637–651.

Ho, Karen. 2005. "Situating Global Capitalisms: A View from Wall Street Investment Banks." *Cultural Anthropology* 20 (1):68–96.

Hogan, Margaret C. et al. 2010. "Maternal Mortality for 181 Countries, 1980–2008: A Systematic Analysis of Progress Towards Millennium Development Goal 5." *Lancet* 375 (9726):1609–1623.

Hong, Y. Y. et al. 2000. "Multicultural Minds—A Dynamic Constructivist Approach to Culture and Cognition." *American Psychologist* 55 (7):709–720.

Horton, R. 2010. "Maternal Mortality: Surprise, Hope, and Urgent Action." *Lancet* 375 (9726):151–2.

Howell, Nancy. 1979. *Demography of the Dobe !Kung*. New York: Academic Press.

Hurtado, Elena. 1984. "Estudio de las Caracteristicas y Practicas de las Comadronas Tradicionales en una Comunidad Indigena de Guatemala." In *Ethnomedicina en Guatemala*, ed. E. M. Villatoro. Guatemala: Centro de Estudios Folkóricos.

———. 1995. *Desde la Comunidad … Percepción de las Complicaciones Maternas y Perinatales y Búsqueda de Atención*. Guatemala: MotherCare USAID MSPAS.

Hymes, Dell. 1973. "Speech and Language: On the Origins and Foundations of Inequality Among Speakers." *Daedalus* 102 (3):59–85.

Inhorn, Marcia Claire. 1994. *Quest for Conception: Gender, Infertility, and Egyptian Medical Traditions*. Philadelphia: University of Pennsylvania Press.

———. 1996. *Infertility and Patriarchy: The Cultural Politics of Gender and Family Life in Egypt*. Philadelphia: University of Pennsylvania Press.

———. 2003. *Local Babies, Global Science: Gender, Religion, and In Vitro Fertilization in Egypt*. New York: Routledge.

Inhorn, Marcia Claire, and Frank van Balen. 2002. *Infertility Around the Globe: New Thinking on Childlessness, Gender, and Reproductive Technologies*. Berkeley: University of California Press.

Instituto Nacional de Estadística. 2002. *Censos 2002: XI de Poblacino y VI de Habitacion*. Guatemala: INE.

Irvine, Judith. 1989. "When Talk Isn't Cheap: Language and Political Economy." *American Ethnologist* 16 (2):248–267.

Jameson, Fredric. 2002. *A Singular Modernity: Essay on the Ontology of the Present*. London, New York: Verso.

Janes, Craig R., and Oyuntsetseg Chuluundorj. 2004. "Free Markets and Dead Mothers: The Social Ecology of Maternal Mortality in Post-Socialist Mongolia." *Medical Anthropology Quarterly* 18 (2):230–257.

Janzen, John M. 1978. *The Quest for Therapy in Lower Zaire, Comparative Studies of Health Systems and Medical Care*. Berkeley: University of California Press.

Jokhio, Abdul Hakeem, Heather R. Winter, and Kar Keung Cheng. 2005. "An Intervention Involving Traditional Birth Attendants and Perinatal and Maternal Mortality in Pakistan." *New England Journal of Medicine* 352 (20):2091–2099.

Jolly, Margaret. 2002. "Birthing Beyond the Confinements of Tradition and Modernity?" In *Birthing in the Pacific: Beyond Tradition and Modernity?* ed. V. Lukere and M. Jolly. Honolulu: University of Hawai'i Press.

Jordan, Brigitte. 1978. *Birth in Four Cultures: A Crosscultural Investigation of Childbirth in Yucatan, Holland, Sweden, and the United States, Monographs in Women's Studies*. Montreal, St. Albans, Vt.: Eden Press Women's Publications.

————. 1989. "Cosmopolitan Obstetrics: Some Insights from the Training of Traditional Midwives." *Social Science Medicine* 28 (9):925–944.

Joseph, Suad. 1994. "Brother/Sister Relationships: Connectivity, Love, and Power in the Reproduction of Patriarchy in Lebanon." *American Ethnologist* 21 (1):50–73.

————. 1996. "Patriarchy and Development in the Arab World." *Gender and Development* 4 (2):14–19.

Justice, Judith. 1986. *Policies, Plans & People: Foreign Aid and Health Development*. Berkeley: University of California Press.

Justus Hofmeyr, G., Lale Say, and A. Metin Gulmezoglu. 2005. "WHO Systematic Review of Maternal Mortality and Morbidity: The Prevalence of Uterine Rupture." *BJOG: An International Journal of Obstetrics and Gynaecology* 112 (9):1221–1228.

Kahneman, Daniel, and Amos Tversky. 1972. "Subjective Probability: A Judgment of Representativeness." *Cognitive Psychology* 3 (3):430–454.

Kasongo Project Team. 1984. "Antenatal Screening for Fetopelvic Dystocia: A Cost-Effectiveness Approach to the Choice of Simple Indicators for Use by Auxiliary Personnel." *Journal of Tropical Medicine and Hygiene* 87(4): 173–183.

Kaspin, Deborah. 1996. "A Chewa Cosmology of the Body." *American Ethnologist* 23 (3):561–578.

Kaunitz, Andrew M., C. Spence, and T. S. Danielson. 1984. "Perinatal and Maternal Mortality in Religious Group Avoiding Obstetric Care." *American Journal of Obstetrics and Gynecology* 150:826–831.

Kennell, John H., et al. 1991. "Continuous Emotional Support During Labor in a United States Hospital—A Randomized Controlled Trial." *Journal of the American Medical Association* 265 (17):2197–2201.

Klaus, Marshal H. et al. 1986. "Effects of Social Support During Parturition on Maternal and Infant Morbidity." *British Medical Journal* 293 (6547): 585–587.

Klein, R. 2000. "From Evidence-Based Medicine to Evidence-Based Policy?" *Journal of Health Service Research and Policy* 5 (2):65–66.

Koblinsky, Marge et al. 2006. "Going to Scale with Professional Skilled Care." *Lancet* 368 (9544):1377–1386.

Kobrak, Paul. 1997. "Village Troubles: The Civil Patrols in Aguacatán, Guatemala." PhD Diss., Department of History, University of Michigan, Ann Arbor.

Kruske, Sue, and Lesley Barclay. 2004. "Effect of Shifting Policies on Traditional Birth Attendant Training." *Journal of Midwifery & Women's Health* 49 (4):306–311.

Kulick, Don. 1992. *Language Shift and Cultural Reproduction: Socialization, Self and Syncretism in Papua New Guinean Village*. Cambridge: Cambridge University Press.

Kwast, Barbara E. 1993. "Safe Motherhood—The First Decade." *Midwifery* 9 (3):105–123.

Labov, William. 1972. *Sociolingusitic Patterns.* Philadelphia: University of Pennsylania Press.

Lawrence, Jane. 2000. "The Indian Health Service and the Sterilization of Native American Women." *American Indian Quarterly* 24 (3):400–419.

Lawrence, Patricia. 2000. "Violence, Suffering, Amman: The Work of Oracles in Sri Lanka's Eastern War Zone." In *Violence and Subjectivity,* ed. V. Das et al. Berkeley: University of California Press.

Leinaweaver, Jessa. 2008. *Circulation of Children: Kinship, Adoption, and Morality in Andean Peru.* Durham: Duke University Press.

Lepri, Isabella. 2005. "The Meanings of Kinship Among the Ese Ejja of Northern Bolivia." *Journal of the Royal Anthropological Institute* 11 (4):703–724.

Lock, Margaret M. 1993. *Encounters with Aging: Mythologies of Menopause in Japan and North America.* Berkeley: University of California Press.

———. 2001. "The Tempering of Medical Anthropology: Troubling Natural Categories." *Medical Anthropology Quarterly* 15 (4):478–492.

Lock, Margaret M., and Judith Farquhar. 2007. *Beyond the Body Proper: Reading the Anthropology of Material Life.* Durham: Duke University Press.

Lock, Margaret M., and Patricia A. Kaufert. 1998. *Pragmatic Women and Body Politics, Cambridge Studies in Medical Anthropology.* New York: Cambridge University Press.

Loudon, Irvine. 1992. *Death in Childbirth: An International Study of Maternal Care and Maternal Mortality, 1800–1950.* Oxford: Clarendon Press.

———. 2000. "Maternal Mortality in the Past and its Relevance to Developing Countries Today." *American Journal of Clinical Nutrition* 72 (1):241S–246S.

MacLeod, Murdo J. 1973. *Spanish Central America: A Socioeconomic History, 1520–1720.* Berkeley: University of California Press.

Madhok, Sumi. 2004. "Heteronomous Women? Hidden Assumptions in the Demography of Women." In *Reproductive Agency, Medicine and the State: Cultural Transformations in Childbearing,* ed. M. Unnithan-Kumar. New York: Berghahn Books.

Mahmood, Saba. 2005. *Politics of Piety: The Islamic Revival and the Feminist Subject.* Princeton: Princeton University Press.

Maine, Deborah, and Allan Rosenfield. 1999. "The Safe Motherhood Initiative: Why Has it Stalled?" *American Journal of Public Health* 89:480–482.

Markowitz, Fran, and Natan Uriely. 2002. Shopping in the Negev: Global Flows and Local Contingencies. *City & Society* XIV (2):211–236.

Martin, Emily. 1992. *The Woman in the Body: A Cultural Analysis of Reproduction.* Boston: Beacon Press.

Maternowska, M. Catherine. 2006. *Reproducing Inequities: Poverty and the Politics of Population in Haiti, Studies in Medical Anthropology.* New Brunswick, NJ: Rutgers University Press.

Maupin, Jonathan Nathaniel. 2008. "Remaking the Guatemalan Midwife: Health Care Reform and Midwifery Training Programs in Highland Guatemala." *Medical Anthropology* 27 (4):353–382.

———. 2009. "'Fruit of the Accords': Healthcare Reform and Civil Participation in Highland Guatemala." *Social Science & Medicine* 68 (8):1456–1463.

Mauss, Marcel. 1985. "Category of the Self." In *The Category of the Person: Anthropology, Philosophy, History*, ed. M. Carrithers, S. Collins, and S. Lukes. Cambridge, New York: Cambridge University Press.

McCreery, David. 1994. *Rural Guatemala, 1760–1940*. Stanford: Stanford University Press.

McDermott, Ray P., and Henry Tylbor. 1995. "On the Necessity of Collusion in Conversation." In *The Dialogic Emergence of Culture*, ed. D. Tedlock and B. Mannheim. Urbana: University of Illinois Press.

Medina-Giron, Haroldo. 1989. *Estudio de Mortalidad Materna en Guatemala: Estimacion de Subregistro*. Guatemala: Ministerio de Salud Pública y Asistencia Social Departamento Materno-Infantil.

Meisch, Lynn A. 1995. "Gringas and Otavaleños: Changing Tourist Relations." *Annals of Tourism Research* 22 (2):441–462.

Menchu, Rigoberta, and Elisabeth Burgos-Debray. 1984. *I, Rigoberta Menchu: An Indian Woman in Guatemala*. London: Verso.

Menéndez, Eduardo L. 1990. *Morir de Alcohol: Saber y Hegemonía Médica*. México City: Alianza Editorial Mexicana, Consejo Nacional para la Cultura y las Artes.

Miller, Suellen et al. 2003. "Where is the 'E' in MCH? The Need for an Evidence-Based Approach in Safe Motherhood." *Journal of Midwifery and Women's Health* 48 (1):10–18.

Milne, Lesley et al. 2004. "Safe Motherhood Program Evaluation: Theory and Practice." *Journal of Midwifery & Women's Health* 49 (4):338–344.

Mohanty, Chandra Talpade, Ann Russo, and Lourdes Torres. 1991. *Third World Women and the Politics of Feminism*. Bloomington: Indiana University Press.

Moraga, Cherríe, and Gloria Anzaldúa. 1983. *This Bridge Called My Back: Writings by Radical Women of Color*. 2nd edition. New York: Kitchen Table, Women of Color Press.

Mosavela, Maghboeba et al. 2005. "Community-Based Participatory Research (CBPR) in South Africa: Engaging Multiple Constituents to Shape the Research Question." *Social Science & Medicine* 61 (12):2577–2587.

MotherCare, and USAID. 1994. *Lograr La Maternidad Sin Riesgo*. Washington, DC: USAID.

MotherCare, USAID, MSPAS, and John Snow, Inc. 1999. *Mortalidad Perinatal en Guatemala: Estudio Comunitario*. Guatemala: USAID.

MSPAS. 2002. *Protocolos de Salud Reproductiva*. Guatemala: MSPAS.

———. 2003. *Línea Basal de Mortalidad Materna Para el Año 2000*. Guatemala: Ministerio de Salud Publica y Asistencia Social.

MSPAS et al. 1996. *Señales de Peligro de Embarazo, Parto y Recién Nacido*. Guatemala: MSPAS.

MSPAS, and MotherCare. 1998. Guia Para el Uso de los Programas de Radio "Salud Para la Vida." Edited by USAID, MotherCare, and J. S. Inc. Guatemala: MSPAS.

MSPAS, MotherCare, and USAID. 1995. *Consejería en el Control Prenatal.* Guatemala.

Mullany, Britta C., Michelle J. Hindin, and Stan Becker. 2005. "Can Women's Autonomy Impede Male Involvement in Pregnancy Health in Katmandu, Nepal?" *Social Science & Medicine* 61 (9):1993–2006.

Nelson, Diane M. 1999. *A Finger in the Wound: Body Politics in Quincentennial Guatemala.* Berkeley: University of California Press.

Nybo, Thomas. 2009. *Fighting Chronic Malnutrition Among Impoverished Children in Guatemala.* UNICEF 2009. http://www.unicef.org/doublepublish/ guatemala_48087.html. Accessed 10 June 2009.

Obermeyer, Carla Makhlouf. 2000. "Risk, Uncertainty, and Agency: Culture and Safe Motherhood in Morocco." *Medical Anthropology* 19 (2):173–201.

Obeyesekere, Gananath. 1992. *The Apotheosis of Captain Cook: European Mythmaking in the Pacific.* Princeton: Princeton University Press.

Ong, Aihwa. 1987. *Spirits of Resistance and Capitalist Discipline: Factory Women in Malaysia, SUNY Series in the Anthropology of Work.* Albany: State University of New York Press.

Ooms, Gorik et al. 2008. "The 'Diagonal' Approach to Global Fund Financing: A Cure for the Broader Malaise of Health Systems?" *Globalization and Health* 4 (1):6.

Ortner, Sherry B. 1989. *High Religion: A Cultural and Political History of Sherpa Buddhism, Princeton Studies in Culture/Power/History.* Princeton: Princeton University Press.

Partnership for Maternal Newborn and Child Health. 2007. *Ten-Year Strategy: The Partnership for Maternal, Newborn and Child Health.* Geneva: World Health Organization.

Paul, Lois. 1975. "Recruitment to a Ritual Role: The Midwife in a Mayan Community." *Ethos* 3:449–467.

Paul, Lois, and Benjamin David Paul. 1975. "The Maya Midwife as Sacred Specialist: A Guatemalan Case." *American Ethnologist* 2 (4):707–726.

Paxson, Heather. 2004. *Making Modern Mothers: Ethics and Family Planning in Urban Greece.* Berkeley: University of California Press.

Paxton, Anne et al. 2005. "The Evidence for Emergency Obstetric Care." *International Journal of Gynecology & Obstetrics* 88 (2):181–193.

Peralta, Gabriel Aguilera, and John Beverly. 1980. "Terror and Violence as Weapons of Counterinsurgency in Guatemala." *Latin American Perspectives* 7 (2/3):91–113.

Petchesky, Rosalind P. 2003. *Global Prescriptions: Gendering Health and Human Rights.* London, New York: Zed Books, in association with United Nations Research Institute for Social Development. Distributed in the USA exclusively by Palgrave.

Pieterse, Jan Nederveen. 1995. "Globalization as Hybridization." In *Global Modernities,* ed. M. Featherstone, S. Lash, and R. Robertson. London: Sage.

Pigg, Stacy Leigh. 1997. "Authority in Translation: Finding, Knowing, Naming, and Training 'Traditional Birth Attendants.'" In *Childbirth and Au-*

thoritative Knowledge: Cross-Cultural Perspectives, ed. R. Davis-Floyd and C. F. Sargent. Berkeley: University of California Press.

———. 2001. "Languages of Sex and AIDS in Nepal: Notes on the Social Production of Commensurability." *Cultural Anthropology* 16 (4):481–541.

Pinto, Sarah. 2008. *Where There is No Midwife: Birth and Loss in Rural India.* New York: Berghahn Books.

Presidencia de la Republica de Guatemala, and Secretaria General de Planificacion. 1996. *Programa del Gobierno de la Republica 1996–2000: Juntos tenemos la oportunidad de transformar Guatemala: Vamos al Cambio.* Guatemala.

Rabinow, Paul. 1996. *Essays on the Anthropology of Reason.* Princeton: Princeton University Press.

Ralstin-Lewis, D. Marie. 2005. "The Continuing Struggle against Genocide: Indigenous Women's Reproductive Rights." *Wicazo Sa Review* 20 (1):71–95.

Rapp, Rayna. 1999. *Testing Women, Testing the Fetus: The Social Impact of Amniocentesis in America, Anthropology of Everyday Life.* New York: Routledge.

Reichard, Gladys A. 1944. *Prayer: The Compulsive Word, Monographs of the American Ethnological Society VII.* New York: Augustin.

Renaudin, P. et al. 2007. "Ensuring Financial Access to Emergency Obstetric Care: Three Years of Experience with Obstetric Risk Insurance in Nouakchott, Mauritania." *International Journal of Gynecology & Obstetrics* 99 (2):183–190.

Rivkin-Fish, Michele R. 2005. *Women's Health in Post-Soviet Russia: The Politics of Intervention, New Anthropologies of Europe.* Bloomington: Indiana University Press.

Rohde, Jon E. 1995. "Removing Risk from Safe Motherhood." *International Journal of Gynecology & Obstetrics* 50 (Supplement 2):S3–S10.

Rosenfield, Allan, and Deborah Maine. 1985. "Maternal Mortality: A Neglected Tragedy; Where is the M in MCH?" *Lancet* 2 (8446):83–85.

Rosenfield, Allan, Deborah Maine, and Lynn Freedman. 2006. "Meeting MDG-5: An Impossible Dream." *Lancet* 368 (9542):1133–1135.

Rosenthal, Caroline. 1987. "Santa Maria de Jesus: Medical Choice in a Highland Guatemalan Town." PhD Diss., Department of Anthropology, Harvard, Cambridge, MA.

Ross, Louise, Padam Simkhada, and W. Cairns S. Smith. 2005. "Evaluating Effectiveness of Complex Interventions Aimed at Reducing Maternal Mortality in Developing Countries." *Journal of Public Health* 27 (4):331–337.

Sangren, P. Steven. 1995. "'Power' Against Ideology: A Critique of Foucaultian Usage." *Cultural Anthropology* 10 (1):3–40.

Sargent, Carolyn F., and Grace Bascope. 1997. "Ways of Knowing About Birth in Three Cultures." In *Childbirth and Authoritative Knowledge: Cross-Cultural Perspectives*, ed. R. Davis-Floyd and C. F. Sargent. Berkeley: University of California Press.

Saunders, Kriemild. 2002. "Introduction: Towards a Deconstructive Post-Development Criticism." In *Feminist Post-Development Thought: Rethinking*

Modernity, Post-Colonialism and Representation, ed. K. Saunders. London: Zed.

Schaumann, Lisa Anne. 1993. "The Impact of Tourism, Development, and Religious Change on the Highland Maya Community of Santa Cruz La Laguna, Lake Atitlan, Guatemala." Masters thesis, Department of Anthropology, Texas A & M University.

Scheper-Hughes, Nancy. 1992. *Death Without Weeping: The Violence of Everyday Life in Brazil.* Berkeley: University of California Press.

———. 1996. "Theft of Life: The Globalization of Organ Stealing Rumors." *Anthropology Today* 12 (3):3–11.

Schieber, Barbara, and Cynthia Stanton. 2000. *Estimación de Mortalidad Materna en Guatemala Período 1996–1998.* Guatemala: GSD Consultores Asociados/Measure/Evaluation Macro International Inc.

Schiller, Nina Glick, Ayse Caglar, and Thaddeus C. Guldbrandsen. 2006. "Beyond the Ethnic Lens: Locality, Globality, and Born-Again Incorporation." *American Ethnologist* 33 (4):612–633.

Schweder, Richard, and Edmund J. Bourne. 1984. "Does the Concept of the Person Vary Cross-Culturally?" In *Culture Theory: Essays on Mind, Self, and Emotion,* ed. R. Schweder and R. LaVine. New York: Cambridge University Press.

Scott, James C. 1985. *Weapons of the Weak: Everyday Forms of Peasant Resistance.* New Haven: Yale University Press.

Seeman, Don. 1999. "'One People, One Blood': Public Health, Political Violence, and HIV in an Ethiopian-Israeli Setting." *Culture Medicine and Psychiatry* 23 (2):159–195.

Shiffman, Jeremy. 2007. "Generating Political Priority for Maternal Mortality Reduction in 5 Developing Countries." *American Journal of Public Health* 97 (5):796–803.

Shiffman, Jeremy, and Ana Lucía Garcés del Valle. 2006. "Political History and Disparities in Safe Motherhood Between Guatemala and Honduras." *Population and Development Review* 32 (1):53–80.

Shiffman, Jeremy, and Stephanie Smith. 2007. "Generation of Political Priority for Global Health Initiatives: A Framework and Case Study of Maternal Mortality." *Lancet* 370 (9595):1370–1379.

Sibley, Lynn, and Theresa Ann Sipe. 2004. "What can a Meta-Analysis Tell us About Traditional Birth Attendant Training and Pregnancy Outcomes?" *Midwifery* 20 (1):51–60.

Silverman, David. 1997. *Discourses of Counseling: HIV Counseling as Social Interaction.* New York: Sage.

Simpson, Bob. 2009. "'Please Give a Drop of Blood': Blood Donation, Conflict and the Haemato-Global Assemblage in Contemporary Sri Lanka." *Body Society* 15 (2):101–122.

Sivaramakrishnan, K. 1995. "Situating the Subaltern: History and Anthropology in the Subaltern Studies Project." *Journal of Historical Sociology* 8 (4):395–429.

Smith, Carol A. 1990a. "Introduction: Social Relations in Guatemala Over Time and Space." In *Guatemalan Indians and the State, 1540 to 1988*, ed. C. A. Smith. Austin: University of Texas Press.

———. 1990b. "The Militarization of Civil Society in Guatemala: Economic Reorganization as a Continuation of War." *Latin American Perspectives* 17 (4):8–41.

———. 1990c. "Origins of the National Question in Guatemala: A Hypothesis." In *Guatemalan Indians and the State, 1540 to 1988*, ed. C. A. Smith. Austin: University of Texas Press.

Smith, Jason B. et al. 2000. "The Impact of Traditional Birth Attendant Training on Delivery Complications in Ghana." *Health Policy Plan* 15 (3):326–331.

Sosa, Roberto et al. 1980. "The Effect of a Supportive Companion on Perinatal Problems, Length of Labor, and Mother–Infant Interaction." *New England Journal of Medicine* 303 (11):597–600.

Spence, C., T. S. Danielson, and Andrew M. Kaunitz. 1984. "The Faith Assembly: A Study of Perinatal and Maternal Mortality." *Indiana Medicine* 77 (3):180–183.

Stack, Carol B. 1974. *All our Kin: Strategies for Survival in a Black Community.* New York: Harper & Row.

Starrs, Ann M. 1998. *The Safe Motherhood Action Agenda: Priorities for the Next Decade.* New York: Family Care International.

———. 2006. "Safe Motherhood Initiative: 20 Years and Counting." *Lancet* 368 (9542):1130–1132.

Strathern, Marilyn. 1988. *The Gender of the Gift: Problems with Women and Problems with Society in Melanesia, Studies in Melanesian Anthropology.* Berkeley: University of California Press.

Street, Alice. 2009. "Failed Recipients: Extracting Blood in a Papua New Guinean Hospital." *Body Society* 15 (2):193–215.

Tannen, Deborah. 1993. *Gender and Conversational Interaction, Oxford Studies in Sociolinguistics.* New York: Oxford University Press.

Taussig, Michael. 1984. "Culture of Terror—Space of Death. Roger Casement's Putumayo Report and the Explanation of Torture." *Comparative Studies in Society and History* 26 (03):467–497.

Tautz, Siegrid et al. 2000. "Between Fear and Relief: How Rural Pregnant Women Experience Foetal Ultrasound in a Botswana District Hospital." *Social Science & Medicine* 50 (5):689–701.

Tedlock, Dennis, and Bruce Mannheim. 1995. *The Dialogic Emergence of Culture.* Urbana: University of Illinois Press.

Thaddeus, Sereen, and Deborah Maine. 1994. "Too Far to Walk: Maternal Mortality in Context." *Social Science & Medicine* 38 (8):1091–1110.

Tita, Alan Thevenet N. 2000. "The Role of Emergency Obstetric Care in the Safe Motherhood Initiative." *American Journal of Public Health* 90 (5):810.

Tita, Alan Thevenet N., et al. 2007. "Two Decades of the Safe Motherhood Initiative: Time for Another Wooden Spoon Award?" *Obstetrics & Gynecology* 110 (5):972–976.

Torpy, Sally J. 2000. "Native American Women and Coerced Sterilization: On the Trail of Tears in the 1970s." *American Indian Culture and Research Journal* 24 (2):1–22.

Trevathan, Wenda. 1987. *Human Birth: An Evolutionary Perspective, Foundations of Human Behavior.* New York: Aldine De Gruyter.

Trouillot, Michel-Rolph. 1990. *Haiti: State Against Nation: The Origins and Legacy of Devalierism.* New York: Monthly Review Press.

Tsing, Anna Lowenhaupt. 2005. *Friction: An Ethnography of Global Connection.* Princeton: Princeton University Press.

Tumin, Melvin Marvin. 1952. *Caste in a Peasant Society: A Case Study in the Dynamics of Caste.* Princeton: Princeton University Press.

Turner, Terence. 1995. "Social Body and Embodied Subject: Bodiliness, Subjectivity, and Sociality Among the Kayapo." *Cultural Anthropology* 10 (2): 143–170.

Turner, Victor. 1957. *Schism and Continuity in African Society.* Manchester: Manchester University Press.

Tversky, A., and D. Kahneman. 1986. "Rational Choice and the Framing of Decisions." *Journal of Business* 59:S251–S278.

Tversky, Amos, and Daniel Kahneman. 1973. "Availability: A Heuristic for Judging Frequency and Probability." *Cognitive Psychology* 5 (2):207–232.

———. 1974. "Judgment Under Uncertainty: Heuristics and Biases." *Science* 185 (4157):1124–1131.

———. 1986. "Rational Choice and the Framing of Decisions." *Journal of Business* 59:S251–S278.

Unnithan-Kumar, Maya. 2004. *Reproductive Agency, Medicine and the State: Cultural Transformations in Childbearing.* New York: Berghahn Books.

Van Hollen, Cecilia. 2003. *Birth on the Threshold: Childbirth and Modernity in South India.* Berkeley: University of California Press.

van Roosmalen, Jos et al. 2005. "Integrating Continuous Support of the Traditional Birth Attendant into Obstetric Care by Skilled Midwives and Doctors: A Cost-Effective Strategy to Reduce Perinatal Mortality and Unnecessary Obstetric Interventions." *Tropical Medicine & International Health* 10 (5):393–394.

Waldrop, Anne. 2004. "Gating and Class Relations: The Case of a New Delhi 'Colony.'" *City & Society* 16 (2):93–116.

Walsh, Julia A., and Kenneth S. Warren. 1980. "Selective Primary Health Care: An Interim Strategy for Disease Control in Developing Countries." *Social Science & Medicine, Part C: Medical Economics* 14 (2):145–163.

Walsh, Linda V. 2006. "Beliefs and Rituals in Traditional Birth Attendant Practice in Guatemala." *Journal of Transcultural Nursing* 17 (2):148–154.

Warren, Kay B. 1998. *Indigenous Movements and Their Critics: Pan-Maya Activism in Guatemala.* Princeton: Princeton University Press.

———. 2001. "Rethinking Bi-Polar Constructions of Ethnicity." *Journal of Latin American Anthropology* 6 (2):90–105.

Weismantel, Mary J. 1995. "Making Kin: Kinship Theory and Zumbagua Adoptions." *American Ethnologist* 22 (4):685–704.

———. 2001. *Cholas and Pishtacos: Stories of Race and Sex in the Andes, Women in Culture and Society.* Chicago: University of Chicago Press.

Williamson, Edwin. 1992. *The Penguin History of Latin America.* London: Allen Lane, The Penguin Press.

Wilson, Ara. 1998. "Decentralization and the Avon Lady in Bangkok, Thailand." *PoLAR: Political and Legal Anthropology Review* 21 (1):77–83.

Wolf, Eric R. 1957. "Closed Corporate Peasant Communities in Mesoamerica and Central Java." *Southwestern Journal of Anthropology* 13 (1):1–18.

Woolard, Kathryn Ann. 1985. "Language Variation and Cultural Hegemony." *American Ethnologist* 12 (4):738–748.

World Bank. 2003. *Guatemala: Poverty in Guatemala.* Washington, DC: World Bank.

World Bank, and International Monetary Fund. 2008. *Global Monitoring Report 2008: MDGs and the Environment: Agenda for Inclusive and Sustainable Development.* Washington, DC: The International Bank for Reconstruction and Development/The World Bank.

World Health Organization. 1995. "Expert Committee Report: Physical Status: The Use and Interpretation of Anthropometry." In *Technical Report Series.* Geneva: World Health Organization.

———. 2005. *World Blood Donor Day: "Celebrating Your Gift of Blood," 14 June 2005: Stories from around the World.* Geneva: World Health Organization.

World Health Organization et al. 2007. *Maternal Mortality in 2005: Estimates Developed by WHO, UNICEF, UNFPA, and the World Bank.* Geneva: World Health Organization.

Yamin, Alicia Ely, and Deborah Maine. 1999. "Maternal Mortality as a Human Rights Issue: Measuring Compliance with International Treaty Obligations." *Human Rights Quarterly* 21 (3):563–607.

SUBJECT INDEX

A

AbouZahr, Carla, 87, 93
Abu-Lughod, Lila, 59
Adams, Richard Newbold, 211n10
Adams, Vincanne, 202n30
agency of women, supporting,
    56–59
Agrawal, Arun, 12–13
agriculture and landholding in
    Santa Cruz, 26–27, 153–55,
    212n23, 213n30
Ahluwalia, Indu B., 207n19
alcohol and alcoholism in Santa
    Cruz, xi, 32–33, 52, 140, 141,
    200n6
Allen, Catherine, 213n26
Allen, Denise Roth, 2, 177, 196n1,
    216n16, 217n18
Alma Ata Conference (1978), Sri
    Lanka, 91, 130, 205n3
Amigos de Santa Cruz, 31
Amnesty International, 138–39
anemia, xii, 7, 73
Annis, Sheldon, 212n23
Anzaldúa Gloria, 209n2
Apffel-Marglin, Frederique,
    202n30
Appadurai, Arjun, 3
Applbaum, Kalman, 3, 197n7
Asowa-Omorodion, Francisca
    Isibhakhome., 102
Atun, Rifat A., 206n8
Augustin, Antoine, 209–10n3

Austin, John L., 202n27
autonomous subjectivity, 192–93
autopsies, xvi–xvii, xviii, 7, 143,
    161, 217n21
Azad, Kishwar, 93

B

Bakhtin, Mikhail, 14
Balen, Frank van, 6
Barclay, Lesley, 84, 89, 91, 100,
    214–15n4
Barnes-Josiah, Debora, 209–10n3
Barnett, Sarah, 93
Bascope, Grace, 196n1
Bastien, Joseph W., 177
Bauman, Richard, 198n17
Becker, Stan, 58
Behague, Dominique P., 92, 205n8
Belaunde, Luisa Elvira, 191
belt used on pregnant women by
    iyoma, xv, 35
"benefits" in Guatemala, 213n27
Bennett, Sara, 206n8
Bernstein, Basil, 61
Berry, Nicole S., 128, 207n23,
    209n8, 210n3, 214n34,
    215n4, 216n14, 217n19
Beverly, John, 211n11
Biehl, João Guilhermo, 5, 14–15,
    197n10
biomedical practice
    empirical knowledge conflicting
        with, 163–66, 169–72

multiple authorities regarding, 166–69
patients' lack familiarity with, 115–17
poverty challenges to, 209–10n3
biomedical workers, *iyoma* distinguished from, 48–56
biomedicalization
    of hunger as sickness, 149–50, 156–57, 158
    of pregnancy, 1–2, 10, 11–12, 61–62, 188–89, 191–92, 196n1
biosocial subjectivities, 5–10, *9, 10,* 188–89, 191–93
birth and birth practices in Santa Cruz, 33–59. *See also* homebirths; hospital and hospital births
    belt used in, xv, 35
    "ideal" birth narrative, 33–36
    illegitimate births, 38–39, 42–45
    kin relationships and, 8–9, *9, 10,* 36–43, 56–57, 59
    risk assessment process and, 39–45
    solitary births, 38–39
    t'uj (sauna), 35, 36, 99–100, 200n10, 207n22
    upright position/husband's support for birth, xv, *10,* 35–36, 59
    women's agency, supporting, 56–59
birth control measures, 180–82, 193
Blaney, David L., 4, 197n8
Bledsoe, Caroline H., 182
blood supply and blood donations, 174–79
Boddy, Janice Patricia, 5
body as indicator of ideologies concerning violence in Guatemala, 140, 150, 159
Bogin, Barry, 158
Bom Jesus, 132, 214n34
book of official acts in hospitals, 117, 119–20

Bourdieu, Pierre, 78
Bourne, Edmund J., 198n12
branding and consolidation of power among evangelicals, 182–83, 217n23
Brass, William, 92
breach births, 168
Briggs, Charles L., 158, 198n17
Brotherton, P. Sean, 14
Brown, Penelope, 61
Bullough, Colin, 93
Burgos-Debray, Elisabeth, 135

C
caesarian and post-caesarean deliveries, 163–66, 174, 179, 180–82, 185
Caglar, Ayse, 197n3
Campbell, Oona, 93, 106, 195, 205n6
Carlough, Martha, 205n5
Carmack, Robert S., 211n11
Carrera, Antonio Goubaud, 211n9
Carsten, Janet, 198n11
Catholicism
    alcohol, views on, 33
    charismatic Catholics, 201n16
    evangelical churches compared, 182, 218n24
CEH (Commission on Historical Clarification), 135
Chapman, Rachel R., 210n3, 216n15, 217n18
Cheng, Kar Keung, 89, 102, 215n4
Chichicastenango, 54, 64, 69, 79
children
    clothing of newborns, 122–24
    fetus, parental attachment to, 111–13
    infant mortality, 52, 80, 86, 113
    jobs and occupations for, 30
    malnourishment and stunting, 147–48, 150, 158
    neglect, doctor's assumption of culture of, 121–22
    schools and schooling, 30–32, 121–22

vaccination of, 148, 215n8
Chimaltenango, 216n13
Chuluundorj, Oyuntsetseg, 2,
    210n3
Chupöl, 61, 68, 69, 79
civil patrols in Guatemala, 132,
    210n4
civil war in Guatemala *(La
    Violencia)*, 95, 132, 134–35,
    139, 181
clothing of newborns, 122–24
Cohen, Lawrence, 181, 217n22
collective ownership, concept of,
    198n13
colonial period and *repartamiento* in
    Guatemala, 133–34
Comaroff, Jean and John, 198n12
Commission on Historical
    Clarification (CEH), 135
Conklin, Beth A., 198n12
contraceptive measures, 180–82,
    193
Cooper, Frederick, 4, 12
Cornwall, Andrea, 209n2
Cosminsky, Sheila, 46, 200n15,
    201n17, 202n26, 209n10
Costello, Anthony, 93
couvade, 191

D
Daniel, Valentine F., 131
Danielson, T. S., 218n26
Das, Veena, 197n10
Davis-Floyd, Robbie, 7–8, 196n1,
    210n3, 216n12
day laborers, 27, 137, 152, 153,
    213n28
de Bernis, Luc, 205n5, 214n4
de León López, Zoila Iris, 214n4
death
    at home versus in hospital, 161
    infant, 52, 80, 86, 113
    maternal. *See* maternal mortality
Delaney, Carol Lowery, 5
Deneux-Tharaux, Catherine, 86,
    92
Donnay, France, 86, 93

doulas in developed world,
    proliferation of, 203n32
Drew, Paul, 61
Duran, Antonio, 206n8
Duranti, Alessandro, 198n17

E
eclampsia and pre-eclampsia, 52,
    53, 89, 119, 191, 201n21
education
    biomedical diagnosis, lack of
        patient familiarity with,
        116–17
    children, schools and schooling
        for, 30–32, 121–22
    midwives, training of, 162, 168,
        214–15n4
    modernity agenda and
        treatment of hospital patients,
        117, 119–21
    teacher-student interaction, 4,
        197n8
    teachers and teaching, 30–32,
        199–200n5
emergency room. *See* hospital and
    hospital births
England, Nora, 211n9
Englund, Harri, 197n3
ER (emergency room). *See* hospital
    and hospital births
"escaping" from hospital, 119–20
Ese Eje, 36
evangelicals
    alcohol, views on, 33, 218n25
    branding and consolidation
        of power among, 182–83,
        217n23
    Catholic Church compared, 182,
        218n24
    daily life in Santa Cruz,
        influence on, 32, 183–84
    homebirths and, 182–87,
        218n26
    identification of indigenous
        dialects and languages by,
        211n19
    illegitimate pregnancies and, 43

iyoma and shamans, 46–47, 53,
    170, 184, 201n17
  number of, 24

F
fainting from blood donation,
    concern over, 177
family. *See* kin relationships
family planning measures, 180–82,
    193
Farmer, Paul, 157, 206n14
farming and landholding in Santa
    Cruz, 26–27, 153–55, 212n23,
    213n30
Farquhar, Judith, 197n9
Fauveau, Vincent, 86, 93
Featherstone, Mike, 196n3
feminism. *See also* women
  agency of women and, 56–59
  birth choice and, 200n8
  status as woman in, 130–31,
    209n2
Ferguson, James, 202n30
fetus, parental attachment to,
    111–13
Figa'-Talamanca, Irene, 207n23
firewood, harvesting and selling,
    28, 171
fishing in Santa Cruz, 27, 27
food access, hunger, and poverty
    in Santa Cruz, 149–53
Forster, Cindy, 139–40
Fortenay, Judith, 92
Foucault, Michel, 6–7, 11–13, 109,
    128–29
Freedman, Lynn P., 90, 106, 205n7
Freire, Paulo, 121, 132
French Revolution, abolition of
    doctors and hospitals after,
    109

G
Gammeltoft, Tine, 120, 191
gangs and gang violence, 138, 139
Garcés del Valle, Ana Lucía, 94,
    102, 210n3
Geertz, Clifforn, 3

geography and topography of
    Santa Cruz, 23–25
Gish, Oscar, 91
Glei, Dana A., 210n3
globalization
  maternal mortality, globalized
    nature of campaign to
    decrease, 196n2. *See also* Safe
    Motherhood campaign
  subjectivity and, 10–15
  theory of, 3–4
Godoy, Angelina Snodgrass, 139,
    212n19
godparents, patronage bond with,
    213n26
Goldman, Noreen, 210n3
Goldstein, Donna, 146
Good, Byron, 5, 14–15, 197n10
Görgen, Regina, 197n4
Graham, Wendy J., 90, 92, 93,
    106, 195, 205n6
Gramsci, Antonio, 132
Grandin, Greg, 212n15, 213n30
Green, Lawrence W., 89
Green, Linda, 131, 132, 208n2,
    210n4, 211n12
gringos in Santa Cruz, 29, 30, 31,
    153–54, 199n3, 213n26
guardianes, 27–28, 153–54, 213n26
Guatemalan State
  blood donation and, 177–78
  civil war in *(La Violencia)*, 95,
    132, 134–35, 139, 181
  globalization and subjectivities,
    14
  labor support research in,
    203n32
  Ministry of Health. *See* Ministry
    of Health
  modernity as agenda for, 108–
    29. *See also* modernity agenda
    and treatment of hospital
    patients
  officials of, group violence
    against, 146–48, 212n20
  Peace Accords (1996), 95, 96,
    107, 135–36, 139, 214n2

Safe Motherhood program, national interpretation of, 4, 13, 86, 94–102, 107
violence as legacy of, 21–22, 130–59. *See also* violence in Guatemala
Guldbrandsen, Thaddeus C., 197n3

H

Hale, Charles R., 208n1, 211n7
Handwerker, Lisa, 197n4
Handy, Jim, 211n10
Hanks, William F., 198n17
Harthorn, Barbara Herr, 217n18
Hastings, Julie A., 211n13
Hay, M. Cameron, 202n24, 210n3, 217n18
hemorrhage, xvi, xvii, 7, 12, 40, 47, 63, 89, 100, 168, 175, 191, 195
high blood pressure, 52, 64, 70, 117–19
Hill, Kenneth, 92
Hindin, Michelle J., 58
Hinojosa, Servando Z., 55
hit-and-run accidents, 145–46
Ho, Karen, 3
Hogan, Margaret C., 206n13, 207n15
homebirths, 22, 160–89
    death at home versus in hospital, 161
    empirical knowledge, biomedical guidelines conflicting with, 163–66, 169–72
    global campaign problematizing, 4
    indigenous preference for, xii, 100, 160–62
    kin relationships and birth practices, ties between, 36–43
    life, valuation of, 160
    midwives' reluctance to make hospital referrals, 162–69
    multiple sources of biomedical information, 166–69

policy changes regarding hospitalization, effects of, 165–66, 168–69
women's agency regarding, 58–59
women's reluctance to go to hospital, 169–86
    blood supply and blood donations, 174–79
    cultural fear of hospital, 172–74
    evangelical churches, influence of, 182–87, 218n26
    operations, concern over, 164–65, 174–82
    Safe Motherhood guidelines and empirical perception of risk, 169–72
Hong, Y. Y., 13
horizontal/vertical policy shifts in Safe Motherhood campaign, 91–93
hospital and hospital births, 21, 60–84
    biomedicalization of pregnancy and, 61–62, 188–89
    blood supply and blood donations, 174–79
    death at home versus in hospital, 161
    doctors and medical specialists, 63–64
    family attendance at, 18–20, 64, 65, 75, 203–4n4
    Guadalupe's experience of, 64–84
        linguistic issues, 76–79, 83–84, 204n6, 204n10–11
        nurse's misrepresentation, 61–62, 67, 73, 81–83, 204n9
        transcript of, 64–76
        transport issues, 79–81, 204n7
    homebirth preferred over. *See* homebirths

"ideal" birth narrative,
interfering with, 40–41
illegitimacy and use of, 44–45
last resort, hospital as, 161–62,
174
layout and procedures of
emergency room, 62–64
modernity, State agenda of,
108–29. *See also* modernity
agenda and treatment of
hospital patients
nurses, 61–62, 63
operations, women's concern
over, 164–65, 174–82
physical access and transport to
hospital, xiii–xv, 62, 79–81,
203n3, 204n7, 209n8
recording procedures, 60–61
reluctance to undergo, xii, xiii,
83
"skilled attendance," privileging
of, 83–84, 89–90, 97–99
women's reluctance regarding.
See under homebirths
household size and structure in
Santa Cruz, 24–25
Howell, Nancy, 33
hunger, food access, and poverty
in Santa Cruz, 149–53
Hurtado, Elena, 96, 207n22
Hymes, Dell, 198n17
hypertension, 52, 64, 70, 117–19

I
IAG (Safe Motherhood Inter-
Agency Group), 87, 89, 90
illegitimate births, 38–39, 42–
45
IMF (International Monetary
Fund), 195
immigration to U.S., 155–56,
214n31
indigenous peoples
evangelical churches,
identification of indigenous
dialects and languages by,
211n19

homebirths, preference for, xii,
100, 160–62
"Indian problem" in Guatemala,
134–36
Indio bruto, concept of, 110–11,
120–28
iyoma, importance of, 194
maternal mortality higher
among, 95, 136
as percentage of Guatemalan
population, 211n9
violence against. *See* violence in
Guatemala
INE (Instituto Nacional de
Estadística), 95
inertia cost, 187
infant mortality, 52, 80, 86, 113
infection, xii, 12, 53, 61, 64, 69,
73, 82–83, 89, 108, 153, 172,
173, 185, 186, 191
Inhorn, Marcia Claire, 3, 6, 202–
3n31, 205n4, 215n5
Instituto Nacional de Estadística
(INE), 95
International Monetary Fund
(IMF), 195
Irvine, Judith, 198n17
iyoma. See midwives

J
Jahn, Albrecht, 197n4
Jameson, Fredric, 109–10, 218n1
Janes, Craig R., 2, 210n3
Janzen, John M., 191
Jhpiego, 97–101, 204n5, 208n3
jobs in Santa Cruz, 27–30, 153–54
John Snow Inc., 96, 98
Johns Hopkins, 97
Jokhio, Abdul Hakeem, 89, 102
Jolly, Margaret, 47, 205n4, 215n5,
216n12
Jordan, Brigitte, 6, 214n3–4
Joseph, Suad, 8–9, 58, 193
justice, crisis of, 137, 138, 142. *See
also* violence in Guatemala
Justice, Judith, 84
Justus Hofmeyr, G., 164

K

Kahneman, Daniel, 217n18
Kaqchikel. *See* indigenous
   peoples
Kaspin, Deborah, 5
Kaufert, Patricia A., 217n17
Kaunitz, Andrew M., 218n26
Kennedy, John F., 3
Kennell, John H., 203n32
K'iche'. *See* indigenous peoples
kidneys, sale of, 181
kin relationships
   birth practices and, 8–9, *9, 10,*
      36–43, 56–57, 59
   birth problems believed to stem
      from, 171, 188, 191
   hospital births, family
      attendance at, 18–20, 64, 65,
      75, 203–4n4
   motherhood and, 190–95
   processual definition of, 8,
      198n11
Klein, R., 89
Kleinman, Arthur, 5, 14–15,
   197n10
Koblinsky, Marge, 93
Kobrak, Paul, 210n4
Kruske, Sue, 84, 89, 91, 100,
   214–15n4
Kulick, Don, 197n6, 198n16
Kwast, Barbara E., 88

L

labor migration, 133–34, 153–56,
   212n24
Labov, William, 61
ladinos, 134, 210–11n7, 213n26
landholding and agriculture in
   Santa Cruz, 26–27, 153–55,
   212n23, 213n30
language. *See* linguistic issues
Lash, Scott, 196n3
Lawrence, Jane, 182
Lawrence, Patricia, 210n5
Leinaweaver, Jessa, 198n11
Lepri, Isabella, 36, 198n11
Levinson, Stephen C., 61

life, valuation of, 113, 160
liminal state, pregnancy as, 22
linguistic issues
   author's learning of Kaqchikel,
      16
   at hospital births, 76–79, 204n6,
      204n10–11
   indigenous dialects and
      languages, 211n9
   interviews and recordings made
      by author, 19–20, 61
   social action, language as, 61,
      198n16–17
Lock, Margaret M., 6, 190, 197n9,
   217n17
Los Encuentros, 79
Loucky, James, 158
Loudon, Irvine, 89
lynchings and threats of lynching,
   139, 146–48, 212n20

M

MacLeod, Murdo J., 210n6
Madhok, Sumi, 59
Mahmood, Saba, 14, 197n10
Maine, Deborah, 87–90, 200n12,
   205n7, 209–10n3
malnourishment and stunting,
   147–48, 150, 158
Mannheim, Bruce, 198n17
maquila jobs, 155
Markowitz, Fran, 197n3
Martin, Emily, 7, 196n1
maternal mortality, 1–22
   biomedicalization of pregnancy
      and, 1–2, 10, 11–12, 61–62,
      188–89, 191–92, 196n1
   biosocial subjectivities and,
      5–10, *9, 10,* 188–89, 191–93
   birth and birth practices,
      33–59. *See also* birth and birth
      practices in Santa Cruz
   death at home versus in
      hospital, 161
   ethnography as means of
      interrupting globalized
      narrative of, 2–4

global campaign to decrease, 21, 85–107. *See also* Safe Motherhood campaign
homebirths, 22. *See also* homebirths
hospital births, 21, 60–84. *See also* hospital and hospital births
indigenous peoples' high rates of, 95, 136
liminal state, pregnancy as, 22
modernity as State agenda and, 21, 108–29. *See also* modernity agenda and treatment of hospital patients
motherhood, importance of emphasizing, 190–96
poverty, special challenges of, 131, 209–10n3
reasons for current global concern with, 106
risk assessment process, 39–45, 88, *88*
Santa Cruz, author's fieldwork in, vii–viii, 15–20, *16, 17*
statistical issues, 86, 92–93, 94–96, 103–4, 206n13
subjectivity and globalization, 10–15
village life and, 20–21, 23–59. *See also* village life
violence and, 21–22, 130–59. *See also* violence in Guatemala
Maternowska, M. Catherine, 207n24, 210n3
Maupin, Jonathan Nathaniel, 129, 206n11, 214n2
Mauss, Marcel, 198n12
Mayan calendar, 47, 200n14
Mayan peoples. *See* indigenous peoples
McCall, Maureen, 205n5
McCreery, David, 146, 211n7–8, 213n30
McDermott, Ray P., 61
MDG (Millennium Development Goals), 90, 194

Médicos del Mundo, 101
Medina-Giron, Heraldo, 94–96
Meisch, Lynn A., 158
Menchu, Rigoberta, 134–35
Menéndez, Eduardo L., 61
Metin Gulmezoglu, A., 164
midwives *(iyoma)*, 45–57
belt used on pregnant women by, xv, 35
biomedical workers, distinguished from, 48–56
choice of, 34–35, 36–37
empirical knowledge, official guidelines conflicting with, 163–66
evangelicalism and, 46–47, 53, 170, 184, 201n17
hospital referrals, reluctance to make, 162–69
importance to indigenous peoples, 194
labor and delivery, assistance with, 35–36, 48, 54
multiple sources of biomedical information for, 166–69
newborn, care of, 36
payment of, 35, 36, 101, 200n11
policy changes regarding hospitalization, reaction to, 165–66, 168–69
pregnancy, role in, 35
reputations of, 171
Safe Motherhood campaign and. *See under* Safe Motherhood campaign
as spiritual practitioners and providers, 45–48, 53–57, 201n17
training of, 162, 168, 214–15n4
vocational aspect of, 45–46
"waiting homes" in Colombia, 207n23
migration, labor-related, 133–34, 153–56, 212n24
migration, to U.S., 155–56, 214n31
Millennium Development Goals (MDG), 90, 194

Miller, Suellen, 89, 93
Milne, Lesley, 93
milpa, 26, 212n23
Ministry of Health. *See also* Sololá
  health workers
  biomedicalization of pregnancy
    by, 189
  blood supply and donations,
    174–75, 177–78
  budget of, 101
  lynching threats against
    malnutrition program, 147–48
  maternal mortality survey,
    94–97
  modernity agenda, 111, 128
  on post-caesarian deliveries, 164
  primary healthcare program
    and, 208n2
  as provider of biomedical
    information to *iyoma,* 166–68
  terms for, 199n18
  tubal ligations and caesarean
    sections, 181–82
MINUGUA (United Nations
  Verification Mission in
  Guatemala), 101, 139, 147
modernity agenda and treatment
  of hospital patients, 21,
  108–29
  biomedical diagnosis, lack of
    patient familiarity with,
    115–17
  book of official acts, 117, 119–20
  choices made for poor by health
    workers, 193–94
  clothing of newborns, 122–24
  defining concepts of modernity,
    109–10
  educating activities, 117, 119–21
  fetus, parental attachment to,
    111–13
  imaginary (modern) patients,
    staff creation of, 111–20
  Indio bruto, concept of, 110–11,
    120–28
  names and naming, local versus
    official, 113–15

non-modern patients, rejection
  of, 108–11
noncompliant patients, 117–20
stereotyping, 121–22
time and timing, 108–10,
  124–28
Western world, association of
  modernity with, 110
Mohanty, Chandra Talpade, 209n2
Molokomme, Imelda, 197n4
Moraga, Cherríe, 209n2
Morgan, Lynn M., 198n12
mortality
  death at home versus in
    hospital, 161
  infant, 52, 80, 86, 113
  maternal. *See* maternal mortality
mo's, 199n3
Mosavela, Maghboeba, 105–6
MotherCare, 96–97
motherhood in maternal mortality,
  importance of emphasizing,
  190–96
MSPAS. *See* Ministry of Health
muchachas, 28, 199n2
Mullany, Britta C., 58
Myntti, Cynthia, 209–10n3

N
Nairobi Conference (1987), 87,
  94, 130
names and naming, local versus
  official, 113–15
Nelson, Diane M., 134
NGOs. *See* nongovernmental
  organizations
noncompliant patients, hospital
  treatment of, 117–20
nongovernmental organizations
  (NGOs). *See also* specific NGOs,
  e.g. Jhpiego
  authority of, 163, 166, 168
  author's fieldwork and, 17
  capacity to provide effective
    care, 119, 129
  coordination with other health
    providers, 102

development programs, funding
for, 207n21
maternal mortality agenda and,
85, 94, 196n2
midwife training by, 168
Nybo, Thomas, 150

O

Oaks, Laury, 217n18
Obermeyer, Carla Makhlouf,
217n17
Obeyesekere, Gananath, 3
obstetric emergency room. *See*
hospital and hospital births
obstructed births, 12, 53, 88, *88*,
89, 191
occupations in Santa Cruz, 27–30,
153–54
Ong, Aihwa, 197n5, 198n15
Ooms, Gorik, 205–6n8
organs, sale of, 181
Ortner, Sherry B., 198n15

P

Panajachel, viii, xiv, *17*, 26, 118,
144, 157, 213n25, 217n23
Partnership for Maternal, Newborn
and Child Health (PMNCH),
90–91
patriarchy, 57–58, 160, 202–3n31
patrilocalism, 34
patronage bond with godparents,
213n26
Paul, Benjamin David, 46
Paul, Lois, 46, 200n13
Paxson, Heather, 192
Paxton, Anne, 205n6
Peace Accords (1996), 95, 96, 107,
135–36, 139, 214n2
Peluso, Daniela, 36
Peralta, Gabriel Aguilera, 211n11
personhood, anthropology of,
198n12
Petchesky, Rosalind P., 206n14
the Petén, vii, 137
Pieterse, Jan Nederveen, 3,
196–97n3

Pigg, Stacy Leigh, 4, 84, 202n30
Pinto, Sarah, 84
pishtacos, 214n32
Pitocin, use of, 12, 167, 168
placenta previa, 178
placental delivery problems, 40,
51, 54, 61, 64, 72, 81, 82, 83,
125, 162, 170, 172, 204n13
Planned Parenthood International,
87
PMNCH (Partnership for Maternal,
Newborn and Child Health),
90–91
police, xvii, 114, 125, 138–46,
209n9, 212n20
Population Council, 87
post-caesarean deliveries, 163–66,
181
pre-eclampsia and eclampsia, 52,
53, 89, 119, 191, 201n21
pregnancy-related death. *See*
maternal mortality
prenatal care, xii, 17, 39–40, 44,
88, 90, 91, 92, 96–97, 130,
192, 210n3
primary healthcare, 87–88, 91,
205n3, 206n10, 208n2
processual definition of kin
relationships, 8, 198n11
prolapsed uterus, 179–80

R

Rabinow, Paul, 5
Ralstin-Lewis, D. Marie, 182
Rapp, Rayna, 7
refrigeration, lack of, 151–52,
212n22
Reichard, Gladys A., 198n17
rejection of non-modern hospital
patients. *See* modernity
agenda and treatment of
hospital patients
relational subjectivities, 57, 58,
191
religion
birth problems and spiritual
challenges, 171

evangelicals. *See* evangelicals
midwives as spiritual
practitioners and providers,
45–48, 53–57, 201n17
Roman Catholic. *See* Catholicism
Renaudin, P., 209n3
repartamiento, 133–34
risk, perception of
at village level, 86–87, 102–6
women's reluctance to go to
hospital and, 169–72
Rivkin-Fish, Michele R., 196n1,
200n8, 208n25
Robertson, Roland, 196n3
Rodriguez, German, 210n3
Rohde, Jon E., 88
Roman Catholicism. *See*
Catholicism
Rosenfield, Allan, 87–90, 205n7
Rosenthal, Caroline, 216n11
Ross, Louise, 205n6
Russo, Ann, 209n2

S
Safe Motherhood campaign, 21,
85–107
biomedicalization of pregnancy
by, 1–2, 10, 11–12, 188–89,
191–92
biosocial subjectivities and, 5–
10, *9, 10,* 188–89, 191–93
cultural orientation of, 7–8
empirical knowledge, guidelines
conflicting with, 163–66,
169–72
ethnography as means of
interrupting globalized
narrative of, 2–4
globalized nature of, 196n2
horizontal/vertical policy shifts,
explaining, 91–93
midwives
empirical knowledge,
guidelines conflicting
with, 163–66
hospital staff reaction to,
100–101

importance of
accommodating, 194–95
incorporation of, 91, 98–102
multiple sources of
biomedical information
for, 166–69
negative views of, 45
training, effectiveness of,
162–63
unskilled biomedical
personnel, treated as, 48,
54–56, 88–89, 202n25–26
national interpretation of, 4, 13,
86, 94–102, 107
official accounts and timeline,
spin provided by, 85–93, 102,
106–7
on post-caesarean deliveries,
163–66, 181
prenatal care, emphasis on, 88,
90, 91, 92, 96–97
risk assessment process, 39–45,
88, *88*
Rosario's story and, 2, 7–8, 11,
16
Santa Cruz, author's fieldwork
in, vii–viii, 15–20, *16, 17*
"skilled attendance," privileging
of, 83–84, 89–90, 97–99, 187,
194–95
SMI agenda, 87–93, 96–98, 195
statistical issues, 86, 92–93, 94–
96, 103–4, 206n13
subjectivity and globalization,
10–15
time and timing in, 125
tubal ligations and caesarean
sections, 181
village-level perception of
maternal mortality and, 86–
87, 102–6
women's agency, nuanced
support of, 57–58
Safe Motherhood Inter-Agency
Group (IAG), 87, 89, 90
San Marcos, *17,* 147–48, 164,
207n22, 212n20

San Pablo, 146–47, 167, 212n18, 212n20

San Pedro La Laguna., *17,* 30–31, 155, 167, 200n13, 212n20

Sanchez, Loyda, 202n30

Sangren, P. Steven, 12

Santa Cruz
  agriculture and landholding in, 26–27, 153–55, 212n23, 213n30
  author's fieldwork in, vii–viii, 15–20, *16, 17*
  birth in. *See* birth and birth practices in Santa Cruz
  food access, hunger, and poverty in, 149–58
  geography and topography, 23–25
  life in. *See* village life
  maternal mortality in. *See* maternal mortality
  tourism in, 29–30, 144–45, 153–54
  water supply and water quality in, 42, 105, 152–53

Santa Elena, 137

Santiago, *17,* 155

Sargent, Carolyn Fishel, 196n1, 216n12

sauna *(t'uj),* 35, 36, 99–100, 200n10, 207n22

Saunders, Kriemild, 58, 202n29

Say, Lale, 164

Schaumann, Lisa Anne, 47

Scheper-Hughes, Nancy, 113, 131, 132, 150, 156–57, 177, 212n19

Schiller, Nina Glick, 197n3

schools and schooling, 30–32, 121–22

Schweder, Richard, 198n12

Scott, James C., 12

Scrimshaw, Mary, 200n15, 209n10

Seeman, Don, 217n22

shamans, xix, 45–47

Sherzer, Joel, 198n17

Shiffman, Jeremy, 92, 94, 102, 210n3

Sibley, Lynn, 89

Silverman, David, 61

Simkhada, Padam, 205n6

Simpson, Bob, 177, 217n22

Sipe, Theresa Ann, 89

Sivaramakrishnan, K., 12

"skilled attendance," privileging of, 83–84, 89–90, 97–99, 187, 194–95

SMI (Safe Motherhood Initiative) agenda, 87–93, 96–98, 195

Smith, Carol A., 134, 211–12n15, 211n7

Smith, Jason B., 89

Smith, Stephanie, 92

Smith, W. Cairns S., 205n6

Snow, Robert W., 92

Sololá. *See* Santa Cruz, and other villages and towns

Sololá health workers
  author's Santa Cruz field work and, vii–viii, 15–20, *16, 17,* 102–3
  globalized program, local/ national interpretation of, 4, 13
  hospital births and. *See* hospital and hospital births
  modernity agenda. *See* modernity agenda and treatment of hospital patients in Rosario's story, xvii, xviii

Safe Motherhood campaign, statistical problems faced by, 92–93, 103

Spence, C., 218n26

spirituality. *See* religion

Stack, Carol B., 202n28

Starrs, Ann M., 88, 89

statistical issues with maternal mortality, 86, 92–93, 94–96, 103–4, 206n13

stereotyping the *Indio bruto,* 121–22

sterilization confused with caesarians, 180–82

Storeng, Katerini T., 92, 205n8
Strathern, Marilyn, 8, 58, 198n12
Street, Alice, 178
student-teacher interaction, 4, 197n8
stunting and malnourishment, 147–48, 150, 158
subjectivities
  autonomous, 192–93
  biosocial, 5–10, *9, 10*, 188–89, 191–93
  globalization and, 10–15
  relational, 57, 58, 191
Summer Institute of Linguistics, 211n9

T
Tannen, Deborah, 61
Taussig, Michael, 131
Tautz, Siegrid, 197n4
teacher-student interaction, 4, 197n8
teachers and teaching, 30–32, 199–200n5
Tecpán, 216n13
Tedlock, Dennis, 198n17
Thaddeus, Sereen, 200n12, 209–10n3
"three delays" framework, 200n12
tiempo, 213n27
Tita, Alan Thevenet N., 93
topography and geography of Santa Cruz, 23–25
Torpy Sally J., 182
Torres, Lourdes, 209n2
tourism in Santa Cruz, 29–30, 144–45, 153–54
transportation
  food access and hunger in Santa Cruz, 151–52, 156, 212n21
  to hospital, xiii–xv, 62, 79–81, 203n3, 204n7, 209n8
transverse pregnancies, 44, 55, 105, 163, 165
trash and trash disposal in Santa Cruz, 25–26
Trevathan, Wenda, 200n7

Trouillot, Michel-Rolph, 131
Tsing, Anna Lowenhaupt, 3
tubal ligations confused with caesarians, 180–82
t'uj (sauna), 35, 36, 99–100, 200n10, 207n22
Tumin, Melvin Marvin, 213n26
Turner, Terence, 197n9
Turner, Victor, 22
Tversky, Amos, 217n18
twins, 42, 168, 216n13
Tylbor, Henry, 61
Tzununá, *17,* 31, 103, 178, 207n21

U
underweight, xii
UNICEF, 150
United Nations, 87, 90, 101
United Nations Verification Mission in Guatemala (MINUGUA), 101, 139, 147
Unnithan-Kumar, Maya, 198n13
upright position/husband's support for birth, xv, *10,* 35–36
Uriely, Natan, 197n3
urinary tract infection (UTI), xii, 64
U.S., immigration to, 155–56, 214n31
USAID, 96, 97
UTI (urinary tract infection), xii, 64

V
vaccinations, 148, 215n8
Van Hollen, Cecilia, 182, 193, 196n1
van Roosmalen, Jos, 102
vertical/horizontal policy shifts in Safe Motherhood campaign, 91–93
vigilantism (lynchings and threats of lynching), 139, 146–48, 212n20
village life, 20–21, 23–59
  agriculture and landholding, 26–27, 153–55, 212n23, 213n30

alcohol and alcoholism, xi, 32–33
birth and birth practices. *See*
   birth and birth practices in
   Santa Cruz
daily routine and timeline, 32
fishing, 27, *27*
geography and topography,
   23–25
gringos, presence of, 29, 30, 31,
   153–54, 199n3, 213n26
household size and structure,
   24–25
jobs and occupations, 27–30,
   153–54
maternal mortality, village-level
   perceptions of, 86–87, 102–6
schooling and education, 30–32
waste and waste disposal, 25–26
violence in Guatemala, 21–22,
   130–59
body as indicator of ideologies
   concerning, 140, 150, 159
civil patrols, 132, 210n4
civil war *(La Violencia)*, 95, 132,
   134–35, 139, 181
class, ethnic, and race-related
   violence, 134–36
colonial period and
   repartamiento, 133–34
community autonomy, efforts to
   break up, 211–12n15
every-day nature of, 131–32,
   157–58
"everything is possible" motto,
   136, 149
food access, hunger, and poverty
   in Santa Cruz, 149–58
gangs, 138, 139
against government officials,
   146–48, 212n20
hit-and-run accidents, 144–46
illegitimate pregnancies
   sparking, 43, 44
"Indian problem" and, 134–36
justice, crisis of, 137, 138, 142
links to maternal mortality, 131,
   132, 136, 158–59
lynchings and threats of
   lynching, 139, 146–48,
   212n20
mayoral candidate, murder of,
   141–42
patriarchy and, 58
payments and bribes, 142–45
Peace Accords (1996), 95, 96,
   107, 135–36, 139, 214n2
police, xvii, 114, 125, 138–46,
   209n9, 212n20
problem of reading/writing
   about, 131, 132–33
protection industry, 137–38
strangers, hesitation to aid,
   144–46
throat-slitting market robberies,
   137
victims, blaming, 137, 138, 139
women, attacks on and by,
   138–41

W
"waiting homes" in Colombia,
   207n23
Waldrop, Anne, 197n3
Walsh, Julia, 206n10
Walsh, Linda V., 46
Wardlaw, Tessa, 93
Warren, Kay B., 211n7, 212n15
Warren, Kenneth, 206n10
waste and waste disposal in Santa
   Cruz, 25–26
water supply and water quality,
   42, 105, 146–47, 152–53
weavers and weaving, *28*, 28–29, *29*
Weismantel, Mary J., 177, 198n11,
   214n32
WHO (World Health
   Organization), 39–40, 42–45,
   87, 89, 90, 96, 150, 179,
   200n8, 205n4
Williamson, Edwin, 210n6
Wilson, Ara, 197n5
Winter, Heather R., 89, 102, 215n4
witchcraft, xviii–xix, 170–71, 188
Wolf, Eric R., 157, 212n15

women. *See also* feminism;
   maternal mortality
   agency of, supporting, 56–59
   homebirths, reasons for
      preferring. *See under*
      homebirths
   jobs and occupations, 28–30
   violence against and by, 138–41
Women Deliver conference (2007),
      130–31, 206–7n15

Woolard, Kathryn Ann, 61
World Bank, 150, 195
World Health Organization
   (WHO), 39–40, 42–45, 87,
   89, 90, 96, 150, 179, 200n8,
   205n4
World Vision, 147

Y
Yamin, Alicia Ely, 88

INDEX TO ETHNOGRAPHIC VIGNETTES

Ada, 177
Alva, 43
Amalia, 216n13
Ana Emiliana, 172–74
Doña Berta, 167
Doña Cecilia, 171
Constancia, 178–79
Consuelo, 123–24
Cristina, 175–77
David, 177
Dinora, 179–80
Eduardo, 175, 176
Elena, 126–28
Fernando, 142–43
Fidelia, 115
Florinda, 169–70
Geronima, 49–53, 201–2n19–21
Doña Gladys, xii, xiii
Guadalupe, 61–62, 64–84,
    204n6–11
Guillermo, 146–47
Doña Inés, xiv, xv, xvi, xvii
Isabel, 179–80
Javiera, 39–40
Jerry, 175–76
Josefa, 37
Julio, xi, xiii, xiv, xvii

Keylor, 177
Laura, 185–86
Lisbeth, 41–42, 56
Lucrecia, 184–86
Luis, 144–45
Marcel, xi–xix
Mercedes, 38–39, 44
Miriam, 111–13
Neli, 55–56, 202n25
Nersa, 49–53
Ofelia, 185–86, 218n27
Petrona, 108–10, 120, 208n1
Ramos, 108–9
Ricarda, 105
Roberto, 142–43
Rosario, xi–xix, 2, 7–8, 11, 16, 33,
    53, 114–15, 161, 170, 171,
    188, 191, 198n14, 207n20,
    217n21
Sandra, 171
Silvia, 117–20, 208–9n6–7
Silvio, xiii, xiv, xv
Sofia, 185, 218n27
Tomasa, 41
Vilma, 44
Yovani, 44

Fertility, Reproduction and Sexuality

Volume 1
Managing Reproductive Life: Cross-Cultural Themes in Fertility & Sexuality
Edited by Soraya Tremayne

Volume 2
Modern Babylon? Prostituting Children in Thailand
Heather Montgomery

Volume 3
Reproductive Agency, Medicine & the State: Cultural Transformations in Childbearing
Edited by Maya Unnithan-Kumar

Volume 4
A New Look at Thai AIDS: Perspectives from the Margin
Graham Fordham

Volume 5
Breast Feeding & Sexuality: Behaviour, Beliefs & Taboos among the Gogo Mothers in Tanzania
Mara Mabilia

Volume 6
Ageing without Children: European & Asian Perspectives on Elderly Access to Support Networks
Philip Kreager & Elisabeth Schröder-Butterfill

Volume 7
Nameless Relations: Anonymity, Melanesia & Reproductive Gift Exchange between British Ova Donors& Recipients
Monica Konrad

Volume 8
Population, Reproduction & Fertility in Melanesia
Edited by Stanley J. Ulijaszek

Volume 9
Conceiving Kinship: Assisted Conception, Procreation & Family in Southern Europe
Monica M. E. Bonaccorso

Volume 10
Where There is No Midwife: Birth & Loss in Rural India
Sarah Pinto

Volume 11
Reproductive Disruptions: Gender, Technology, & Biopolitics in the New Millennium
Edited by Marcia C. Inhorn

Volume 12
Reconceiving the Second Sex: Men, Masculinity, & Reproduction
Edited by Marcia C. Inhorn, Tine Tjørnhøj-Thomsen, Helene Goldberg & Maruska la Cour Mosegaard

Volume 13
Transgressive Sex: Subversion & Control in Erotic Encounters
Edited by Hastings Donnan & Fiona Magowan

Volume 14
European Kinship in the Age of Biotechnology
Edited by Jeanette Edwards & Carles Salazar

Volume 15
Kinship & Beyond: The Genealogical Model Reconsidered
Edited by Sandra Bamford & James Leach

Volume 16
Islam and New Kinship: Reproductive Technology & the Shariah in Lebanon
Morgan Clarke

Volume 17
Midwifery & Concepts of Time
Edited by Chris McCourt

Volume 18
Assisting Reproduction, Testing Genes: Global Encounters with the New Biotechnologies
Edited by Daphna Birenbaum-Carmeli & Marcia C. Inhorn

Volume 19
Kin, Gene, Community: Reproductive Technologies among Jewish Israelis
Edited by Daphna Birenbaum-Carmeli & Yoram S. Carmeli

Volume 20
Abortion in Asia: Local Dilemmas, Global Politics
Edited by Andrea Whittaker

Volume 21
Unsafe Motherhood: Mayan Maternal Mortality & Subjectivity in Post-War Guatemala
Nicole S. Berry

Volume 22
Fatness & the Maternal Body: Women's Experiences of Corporeality & the Shaping of Social Policy
Edited by Maya Unnithan-Kumar & Soraya Tremayne

Volume 23
Islam & Assisted Reproductive Technologies: Sunni & Shia Perespectives
Edited by Maria C. Inhorn & Soraya Tremayne

Volume 24
Militant Lactivism? Infant Feeding & Maternal Accountability in the UK & France
Charlotte Faircloth

CPSIA information can be obtained
at www.ICGtesting.com
Printed in the USA
JSHW011418241019
2055JS00008B/96

9 780857 457912